ARCO

MASTER THE

PCAT®

9th Edition

ARCO

MASTER THE

PCAT®

9th Edition

Dick R. Gourley
B.S.Ph., Pharm.D.
Greta A. Gourley
B.S.N., M.S.N., Pharm.D., Ph.D.

THOMSON
PETERSON'S

Australia • Canada • Mexico • Singapore • Spain • United Kingdom • United States

An ARCO Book

ARCO is a registered trademark of Thomson Learning, Inc., and is used herein under license by Peterson's.

About The Thomson Corporation and Peterson's

With revenues of US$7.8 billion, The Thomson Corporation (www.thomson.com) is a leading global provider of integrated information solutions for business, education, and professional customers. Its Learning businesses and brands (www.thomsonlearning.com) serve the needs of individuals, learning institutions, and corporations with products and services for both traditional and distributed learning.

Peterson's, part of The Thomson Corporation, is one of the nation's most respected providers of lifelong learning online resources, software, reference guides, and books. The Education Supersite^{SM} at www.petersons.com—the Internet's most heavily traveled education resource—has searchable databases and interactive tools for contacting U.S.-accredited institutions and programs. In addition, Peterson's serves more than 105 million education consumers annually.

For more information, contact Peterson's, 2000 Lenox Drive, Lawrenceville, NJ 08648; 800-338-3282; or find us on the World Wide Web at: www.petersons.com/about

ISSN: International Standard Serial Number information available upon request.

ISBN: 0-7689-2228-3

Printed in the United States of America

10 9 8 7 6 5 4 3 2 1   07 06 05

Ninth Edition

Contents

Before You Begin ix

How This Book Is Organized ix
Special Study Features x
You're Well On Your Way to Success x
Top 10 Ways to Raise Your Score xi

PART I: PCAT BASICS

1   All About the PCAT 3

When to Take the PCAT 4
How Many Times Should I Take the PCAT? 4
How the Test Is Scored 4
Applying for the Test 5
At the Test Center 10
Test Content 11
PCAT Study Plan 26
Summing It Up 27

PART II: DIAGNOSING STRENGTHS AND WEAKNESSES

2   Practice Test 1: Diagnostic 39

Answer Key and Explanations 90

PART III: PREPARING FOR YOUR PHARMACY CAREER

3   Pharmacy Education 135

Accreditation of Pharmacy Education 135
Institutions and Programs 136
Pharmacy Students 136
Components of Pharmacy Education 137
Degrees Offered 137
Pre-Pharmacy Requirements 138
Professional Pharmacy Curriculum 141
Frequently Asked Questions About Pharmacy Education 144
Summing It Up 146

4   Admission Process **147**

Requirements for Admission 147
Health Profession Advisers 148
Application Process 148
Pharmacy Education Costs 149
Financial Aid 149
Summing It Up 151

5   Postgraduate Education **153**

Residencies 153
Frequently Asked Questions About Pharmacy Residencies 153
Fellowships 156
Graduate Education 156
Summing It Up 157

6   Making Pharmacy Your Career **159**

Career Opportunities 159
Pharmacist Responsibilities for Patient-Centered
   Pharmaceutical Care 163
Factors Affecting the Pharmacy Profession 164
Summing It Up 165

PART IV: PRACTICE TEST

Practice Test 2 .... **177**

Answer Key and Explanations 215

APPENDIXES

A   AACP Member Colleges and Schools of Pharmacy **239**

B   State Boards of Pharmacy **257**

C   Licensure Requirements **269**

Before You Begin

HOW THIS BOOK IS ORGANIZED

The standard dictionary definition of *pharmacy* is "the art or practice of preparing, preserving, compounding, and dispensing drugs." These were the traditional roles of the pharmacist. However, career opportunities in pharmacy are much broader today and range from storing and purchasing medications to education to specialty pharmacy practice (e.g., geriatrics, pediatrics, oncology, or nuclear pharmacy).

Technology has made a dramatic difference in the provision of health care. Likewise, the role of the pharmacist as a health-care professional has expanded with the development of the pharmaceutical care movement.

To prepare future pharmacists for these expanded roles, pharmacy education has moved from a chemistry/laboratory-based education to a more biological/practice-based education, and students need to prepare for these changing responsibilities. *ARCO Master the PCAT* provides you with the necessary ammunition to help you prepare for the PCAT and a career in pharmacy, including:

"Top 10 Ways to Raise Your Score" gives you a preview of some of the test-taking strategies you'll learn in the book.

Part I provides essential information about the PCAT including how to register for the test, test content, and proven test-taking strategies.

Part II is a full-length diagnostic test, which is your first chance to work with samples of every PCAT question type. It can show you where your skills are strong and where they need some shoring up.

Part III provides you with the ins and outs of pharmacy education, the admission process, postgraduate education, and career opportunities.

Part IV is a full-length practice test followed by detailed answer explanations for each question.

The **Appendixes** contain information about licensure requirements, a directory of accredited colleges and schools of pharmacy, and state boards of pharmacy.

SPECIAL STUDY FEATURES

ARCO Master the PCAT is designed to be as user-friendly as it is complete. To this end, it includes several features to make your preparation much more efficient.

Overview

Each chapter begins with a bulleted overview listing the topics that will be covered in the chapter. This will allow you to quickly target the areas in which you are most interested.

Summing It Up

Each chapter ends with a point-by-point summary that captures the most important points contained in the chapter. They are a convenient way to review key points.

As you work your way through the book, keep your eye on the margins to find bonus information and advice. Information can be found in the following forms:

Note

Notes highlight critical information about the PCAT and a career in pharmacy.

Tip

Tips draw your attention to valuable concepts and advice for tackling the PCAT.

Alert!

Alerts do just what they say—alert you to common pitfalls or misconceptions.

YOU'RE WELL ON YOUR WAY TO SUCCESS

You have made a decision to pursue a career in pharmacy. *ARCO Master the PCAT* will prepare you for the steps you'll need to take to achieve your goal—from scoring high on the PCAT to choosing a career path best suited for you. Good luck!

Top 10 Ways to Raise Your Score

The following strategies are suggested to help you do your best on the PCAT:

1. **Familiarize yourself with the test.** Review the test content and take the practice test in this book under timed conditions.

2. **Because most of the test involves knowledge, skills, and abilities accumulated over time, cramming probably will not help much.**

3. **Be prepared physically and mentally.** Get a good night's sleep the night before your test, eat what you consider a normal meal the morning of the test, and dress comfortably for the test.

4. **On the day of the test, dress in a manner that will allow you to adapt to different room temperatures.**

5. **Allow plenty of time to get to your Test Center.**

6. **Answer as many questions as time allows.** There is no penalty for guessing, so it is to your advantage to answer every question.

7. **When you are not sure which answer choice is correct, eliminate as many incorrect options as you can.** When you have doubts about an answer to a question, change your answer only if you have a valid reason.

8. **Do not dwell on items that are unfamiliar or difficult, since all the questions count the same.** In each of the first five multiple-choice subtests, first answer questions about which you are confident, and then return to answer the more difficult items if time permits.

9. **Work quickly but carefully.**

10. **Check regularly to make sure you are marking your answers in the correct place on the answer sheet.**

PART I

PCAT BASICS

CHAPTER 1   All About the PCAT

All About the PCAT

OVERVIEW

- **When to take the PCAT**
- **How many times should I take the PCAT?**
- **How the test is scored**
- **Applying for the test**
- **At the test center**
- **Test content**
- **PCAT study plan**
- **Summing it up**

The Pharmacy College Admission Test (PCAT), an exam developed by PsychCorp, a brand of Harcourt Assessment, Inc., is a specialized test that helps identify qualified applicants to pharmacy colleges. It measures general academic ability and scientific knowledge necessary for the commencement of pharmaceutical education. The PCAT is constructed specifically for colleges of pharmacy. The test is generally given three times a year in October, November, and January.

The American Association of Colleges of Pharmacy (AACP) endorses the PCAT as the official preferred admission test for entrance to pharmacy college.

Direct all requests for information concerning the PCAT and requests for special services to the following address:

Harcourt Assessment, Inc.
PSE Customer Relations — PCAT
19500 Bulverde Road
San Antonio, TX 78259
Phone: (800) 622-3231
Fax: (888) 211-8276
Web site: www.pcatweb.info
E-mail: Scoring.Services@Harcourt.com

chapter 1

WHEN TO TAKE THE PCAT

Find out the deadline for completion of the applications for the college/school(s) of pharmacy in which you are interested. Allow yourself plenty of time to meet the deadlines. Do not wait until the last possible test date to take the PCAT.

It is recommended that you take the PCAT the first time it is offered. Therefore, if you have a low score, you can take the examination again and improve your score. Even if the school that you think you will be going to does not require the PCAT, it would be wise to take the examination in case you change your mind about the school/college to which you are applying.

Try to take the PCAT at least two to three test dates before the deadline for your completed admission portfolio in case you need to take the examination again before the school(s) admissions deadline. This is an important strategy to remember, because it will give you a chance to improve your score, if needed.

HOW MANY TIMES SHOULD I TAKE THE PCAT?

The number of times you should take the PCAT depends on your score. If your score meets the criteria for the school(s) to which you are applying and you are satisfied with the score, then you do not need to take the PCAT again. However, if your score does not meet the admissions criteria of the school(s) to which you have submitted applications, then you need to take the examination again.

Here are four factors involved in how many times you take the PCAT:

1. Your percentile score
2. If your score meets the admissions requirements of the school(s) where you have submitted applications
3. When you have taken enough pre-pharmacy courses to feel confident about taking the PCAT
4. If the school(s) to which you have submitted applications consider only the *highest* PCAT score, then take the PCAT until you are satisfied with your score.

HOW THE TEST IS SCORED

Approximately four to five weeks following the date of testing, you will be sent your personal Score Report, and the institutions to which you requested your scores be reported will be sent official transcripts. Under no circumstances will scores be reported over the phone or faxed.

Do not attempt to send copies of your personal Score Report to schools to which you are applying. Schools will only accept official transcripts. Any other PCAT scores you have earned during the previous five years also will be reported on your official transcripts, unless you selected the "No Score Option." Scores more than five years old will not be reported.

When you receive your Score Report, your scores will be reported as scaled scores and percentiles for each of the five multiple-choice subtests and for the multiple-choice test as a whole (Composite). You also will receive a separate score for the Writing subtest.

Different forms of any test may vary somewhat in difficulty. Because of the differences in difficulty between different forms of the PCAT, the same raw scores on different forms are not necessarily equivalent. Using the statistical process of equating, it is possible to express scores in comparable terms across different forms of the test. Scaled scores are used for this purpose. The scale used for the PCAT ranges from 200 to 600, with a median of 400 (i.e., a scaled score of 400 corresponds to the 50th percentile). Raw scores for the Writing subtest range from one to five.

In addition to scaled scores, your personal Score Report will list five subtest percentiles and a Composite percentile. The percentile score shown on your personal Score Report indicates the percentage of PCAT examinees that made up the norm group—all first-time examinees who took the test between October 1998 and March 2003—with scaled scores lower than yours. For example, an examinee who earns a Composite percentile score of 70 scored higher than 70 percent of the examinees from the norm group on the test as a whole.

There is no passing or failing score for this test. The extent to which test results are used in deciding whether or not a person will be admitted to a college of pharmacy varies from one school to another. In general, test results are combined with other information, such as high school and undergraduate records, references, and the results of personal interviews.

TIP

Please consult the schools to which you are applying for information about their use of test scores.

The No Score Option

During the test, you will be able to request that your test not be scored. Before the test begins, the examiner will explain how to request that your test not be scored. Choosing the No Score Option means that scores will not be released to you or to any schools you request. If you request that your test not be scored, the request is irrevocable, and the fees you paid will not be refunded. Any later requests to score your test and report your scores will not be honored.

APPLYING FOR THE TEST

To register for the PCAT, you must complete a paper or online application and submit it with your fee payment by the appropriate application deadline.

If you submit a paper application and it is received after the non-standard application deadline, you will not be registered, and the application deadline will not be extended.

You cannot take the PCAT as a "standby" candidate by showing up at a test center without being registered in advance. There is no late application deadline for paper applications.

Applying Online

You can ensure that your application and payment are received immediately by registering online at www.PCATweb.info. You will find complete instructions online for submitting an application electronically.

You may register online between the standard application deadline and the late application deadline. However, this requires a late fee in addition to the online application fee. A late application is possible only if you register online.

Once you have registered online, do not send in a paper application. Do not register both ways or your application will be delayed and you will be subject only to a partial refund.

Tips for Applying

- **Choose a test date that will ensure that each institution to which you are applying will receive your scores before its application deadline.** Score Reports are mailed approximately four to five weeks after each test date.
- **Apply early.** Paper applications must be received by the paper application deadline. You may want to use an overnight courier service if you are submitting a paper application by mail close to a deadline. If your paper application and fee payment are received after the deadline, you will receive a partial refund.
- **In order to take the PCAT, you must register prior to the deadline for the desired test date.** There will be no opportunity to take the PCAT as a standby.
- **Complete all the information required in your application.** Only properly completed applications will be accepted.
- **If you submit a paper application, sign (do not print) your signature in the space requested.** Unsigned applications will not be accepted. If applying online, a "signature" checkbox must be selected.
- **Include a money order payable to Harcourt Assessment, Inc., with your paper application.** Personal checks will not be accepted. Do not send cash. If personal checks or cash are sent as payment for fees, the accompanying application will not be processed and you will receive only a partial refund.
- **If you are applying online, payment must be made with a credit card.**

The Admission Ticket

Whether you apply online or submit a paper application, within 48 hours after your application is received and processed, you will receive an electronic registration confirmation notice with information about your Admission Ticket. This notice will be sent to the e-mail address that you provide on your application. Approximately 10 days before your PCAT test date, you will receive another e-mail message with instructions on how to access and print your Admission Ticket.

The Admission Ticket shows the complete reporting address of the Test Center that you requested, the exact time that you should report to the Test Center, and an assigned candidate ID number. When you report to the Test Center, you must present your Admission Ticket to gain admittance. If you do not attend your assigned Test Center on the correct test date or do not have your Admission Ticket, you will not be able to take the test, and the fees you paid will not be refunded.

Application Fees and Special Services

If you apply online, you must pay with a credit card. Your fee payment will be received immediately upon electronic submission.

If you submit a paper application, you must pay with a money order. Your money order must display your name. Make your money order payable to Harcourt Assessment, Inc. If you are applying from outside the U.S., you must submit an international money order payable in U.S. dollars. Do not send cash or personal checks.

All PCAT fee payments are deposited immediately upon receipt. However, the deposit of your fee payment does not guarantee that you will be admitted to the test.

PCAT Fees

Online registration fee: $105.00

Paper application fee: $125.00

Duplicate score report fee: $20.00

Test Fee: $105.00 for online registration; $125.00 for a paper application

Optional Fees

Late online application fee: To apply online after the standard application deadline, but before the late application deadline, you must pay $49.00 in addition to the test fee. Remember that if you submit a paper application, your application and fee payment must be received by the non-standard application deadline.

Special testing location fees ($189.00 plus administrative fees for outside U.S./ $189.00 for inside U.S.): Special testing locations for the established testing dates may be arranged for candidates living more than 150 miles from a scheduled Test Center. If you wish to request a special testing location within the U.S., Harcourt Assessment must receive your application, fee payment, and written request for a special testing

ALERT!

A late paper application will not be accepted.

location by the non-standard application deadline. The fee payment is nonrefundable. You may submit this written request when registering online at the PCAT Web site. If you are submitting a paper application, you must mail your request along with your application. If you require a special testing location in a country other than the U.S., call PSE Customer Relations at (800) 622-3231 for additional information.

Whether applying online or with a paper application, to request a special testing location you must submit the following:

1. A completed application and the test fee payment
2. The special testing location fee payment
3. A written explanation to Harcourt Assessment
4. For foreign locations—the name, country, telephone number, and e-mail address of the university

Although Harcourt Assessment cannot guarantee that the PCAT will be administered at the testing location you prefer, every attempt will be made to have it administered at your preferred location or within 75 miles of the address at which you will be residing on the test date for which you are applying. No arrangements for a Special Testing Location will be made unless your application, written request, and the entire fee payment have been received by the non-standard application deadline.

Additional transcript fee: You must pay the additional transcript fee of $20.00 for each official transcript beyond the three that your test fee covers and for any requested after you submit your application.

Canceling Your Registration

If you know you will not be able to take a test for which you have already registered, you may request a cancellation of your registration. You may be able to receive a partial refund if your request for cancellation is received by Harcourt Assessment before the registration cancellation deadline for the appropriate test date. Cancellations received after the posted deadline will not be eligible for any refund.

If you registered online, you must cancel your registration online. If you submitted a paper application, you must request cancellation by writing to Harcourt Assessment. Your written cancellation request must include the following:

1. Your name, address, and Social Security number
2. The name of the test you are registered to take—PCAT
3. The date you are scheduled to test
4. Your signature
5. Your original admission ticket (not a photocopy)

You can mail your cancellation request to:

Harcourt Assessment, Inc.
PSE Customer Relations—PCAT
19500 Bulverde Road
San Antonio, TX 78259
Fax: (888) 211-8276

Non-Saturday Administrations

For candidates whose religious convictions prohibit them from testing on a Saturday, a special testing date may be arranged. There is no additional fee for a non-Saturday test administration. At the time of registration (either online or with a paper application), you will indicate your need for a special arrangement, but your actual request for a non-Saturday administration must be made in writing and submitted by mail and received by Harcourt Assessment by the non-standard application deadline. A non-Saturday administration is generally given on the Sunday or Monday immediately following the Saturday test date.

Your written request must include the following in one complete package:

1. A cover letter specifying that a non-Saturday administration is needed
2. A letter on letterhead from your rabbi, pastor, or religious leader in support of your request for a non-Saturday test date

If you are submitting a paper application, you must include the cover letter and the letter from your religious leader along with the completed paper application and fee payment.

Mail the cover letter and the letter from your religious leader to:

Harcourt Assessment, Inc.
PSE Customer Relations—PCAT
19500 Bulverde Road
San Antonio, TX 78259
Fax: (888) 211-8276

Accommodations for Candidates with Disabilities

Requests for accommodations for candidates with disabilities must be received by Harcourt Assessment by the non-standard application deadlines. There is no additional charge for special accommodations for candidates with disabilities. At the time of registration (either online or with a paper application), you will indicate your need for a special arrangement, but your actual request for special accommodations must be made in writing and submitted by mail.

Your written request must include the following in one complete package:

1. A completed Accommodations Request Form, found online at the PCAT Web site.

2. A current letter (not more than three years old) from a licensed physician, school official, licensed psychologist, or other appropriate authority (a licensed professional whose training is applicable to diagnosis of the disability) on his or her letterhead that includes the licensed professional's title, address, and telephone number; a description of the nature of the functional limitation as it applies to taking a multiple-choice standardized test; and the specific accommodations you will need for testing.

Mail the Accommodations Request Form and letter from the licensed professional to:

Harcourt Assessment, Inc.
PSE Customer Relations—PCAT
19500 Bulverde Road
San Antonio, TX 78259
Fax: (888) 211-8276

AT THE TEST CENTER

Test Day Schedule

- Students are to arrive at the Test Center no later than 8:30 a.m.
- Testing ends at approximately 1:30 p.m.
- In some circumstances, high-volume Test Centers have to schedule both morning and afternoon sessions. You will be notified if you are assigned to an afternoon session.

Test Center Rules

- Take several sharpened number 2 pencils with erasers to your Test Center. For accurate scoring of your answer sheet, only number 2 pencils can be used. Mechanical pencils, ink pens, felt-tip pens, or ballpoint pens cannot be used.
- You must take your Admission Ticket to the Test Center.
- You must take two forms of identification to your Test Center including one with a photograph and signature, such as a driver's license, school identification card, government-issued identification card, or passport. Photo ID credit cards, however, are not acceptable. A second form of positive identification may include a Social Security card, birth certificate, credit card, library card, or utility bill with your name and address.
- You must arrive at your Test Center on time. Testing will begin promptly. Late arrivals will not be admitted.
- If you report to a center other than the one to which you were assigned, or if you do not take your Admission Ticket with you to the Test Center, you will not be able to take the PCAT. Test Centers will not admit standby candidates to take the PCAT.

- At 8:30 a.m., registered candidates will be admitted to the testing room. No candidate will be admitted to the testing room after the test has begun.

- You may not take calculators (including watch calculators), books, papers, notes, pagers, PDAs, cellular phones, recording devices, or any other electronic devices or reference materials into the testing room. You will be allowed to write in your test booklet.

- Neither food nor beverages may be taken into the testing room.

- Visitors are not allowed in the testing room.

- You may not ask questions about the test after the test has begun.

- There will be a rest break approximately halfway through the test. Any examinee who leaves the testing room before or after the break must first receive permission from the examiner and will be escorted while outside the testing room.

- Candidates are prohibited from removing any testing materials from the testing room. This will result in the cancellation of your scores.

- Any candidate who gives or receives assistance during the test will be required to turn in all test materials immediately and leave the room. In such a case, the candidate's answer sheet will not be scored, and no fee payments will be refunded to the candidate.

TEST CONTENT

The PCAT consists of approximately 280 multiple-choice questions. Each question has four answer choices listed, only one of which is correct. The answer to each question can be determined independently of the answers to any other question.

You will have approximately four and one-half hours to complete the test (not including a short rest break about halfway through the test). The PCAT is divided into separate sections, or subtests, each of which is timed separately.

During the time allowed for each subtest, you will be permitted to work only on that section. You will not be allowed to go back to earlier subtests or on to later ones. As you work on each section, you may find it useful to first answer the questions that are easy for you, skipping over those questions to which you will need to return for further thought.

There are six content areas measured by the PCAT in six separate subtests:

- The **Verbal Ability** section measures general, non-scientific word knowledge and usage using analogies and sentence completion.

- The **Quantitative Ability** section measures skills in mathematical processes and the ability to reason through and understand quantitative concepts and relationships, including applications of algebra, geometry, probability and statistics, pre-calculus, and calculus.

- The **Biology** section measures knowledge of the principles and concepts of basic biology, including general biology, microbiology, and human anatomy and physiology.

ALERT!

The order in which the sections are arranged on the actual PCAT may not be the same as is in this book. The order of the sections change with different examinations and dates.

- The **Chemistry** section measures knowledge of principles and concepts of inorganic and elementary organic chemistry.
- The **Reading Comprehension** section measures ability to comprehend, analyze, and evaluate reading passages on science-related topics.
- The **Critical Thinking Essay** section measures conventions of language and composition skills in a written essay. There is one essay topic in this section that requires you to write either an argumentative or problem-solving essay.

The following chart indicates the number of questions per section and the time allowed for each.

NOTE

The form of the PCAT that you take may contain experimental multiple-choice items that are embedded within the first five subtests. The experimental items are being tried out for future use on PCAT test forms and will not affect your score.

Section	Number of Questions	Time
Verbal Ability	58	35 Minutes
Quantitative Ability	58	50 Minutes
Biology	58	35 Minutes
Chemistry	58	35 Minutes
Reading Comprehension	48	50 Minutes
Critical Thinking Essay	N/A	30 Minutes

Verbal Ability

Communication skills are important to the pharmacy profession, enabling pharmacists to provide comprehensive care to patients and to communicate effectively with other health-care providers. The ability to clearly express verbal and written thoughts is a desirable attribute for pharmacists. Many colleges/schools of pharmacy evaluate communication skills during the admissions interview. For example, the admissions committee may ask you to write a brief answer to a question or to write on a specific topic during the interview. The Verbal Ability section measures general, non-scientific word knowledge and usage using analogies and sentence completion.

Quantitative Ability

TIP

Because the test is timed, review all of the relevant topics in the Quantitative Ability section ahead of time to work as quickly as possible.

The PCAT Quantitative Ability section measures skills in mathematical processes and the ability to reason through and understand quantitative concepts and relationships, including applications of algebra, geometry, probability and statistics, pre-calculus, and calculus. You will encounter word problems and also equations to simplify and solve.

When solving problems involving units, it is prudent to write down the units along with the values of the variables to ensure that your final calculated result has the correct units (e.g., grams, centimeters, and gallons).

Biology

The ultimate goal of pharmaceutical care is to optimize therapeutic outcomes, i.e., reduce the incidence of adverse side effects while at the same time increasing drug efficiency via individualization of drug therapy. To this end, a pharmacist must understand how drugs act on the body (pharmacology), how the body acts on drugs (pharmacokinetics), and how disease (pathophysiology) affects a drug's pharmacology and pharmacokinetics.

To be prepared for the academic rigors of pharmacy school, you must have a good background in the disciplines of cellular and molecular biology, anatomy and physiology, and biochemistry. In fact, studies have shown that a student's performance on the Biology section of the PCAT is a good predictor of academic success in pharmacy school. Below is a breakdown of the major points you will need to know for the Biology section of the PCAT:

1) **Molecular Cell Biology**
   a) All animal cells are composed of a cell membrane, cytoplasm, cytoplasmic organelles, and a nucleus.
   b) Fluid Mosaic Model
   c) Integral proteins are intimately associated with the membrane lipids and cannot be extracted from the membrane without membrane disruption.
   d) Membrane proteins are located on the cytoplasmic surface of the cell and are associated with cell shape and motility.
   e) Cytoplasmic organelles
   f) Membrane transport
   g) Cell cycle
   h) Cellular respiration
   i) Molecular biology
2) **Organ Systems**
   a) Tissue organization
      i) The four major types of tissue include epithelial, connective, muscle, and nervous.
      ii) Extracellular fluid is composed of interstitial fluid and plasma.
      iii) The three types of cell junctions include tight junctions, desmosomes, and gap junctions.
      iv) Exocrine glandular secretions
   b) Skeletal system
      i) Function: support, protection of underlying organs, movement, mineral and energy storage, and hematopoiesis
      ii) Organs: bones, tendons, ligaments, and cartilage

  c) Muscular system
    i) Function: locomotion and manipulation, vision, facial expression (skeletal), blood pumping (cardiac), food digesting, urination (smooth), posture, joint stability, and heat generation
    ii) Organs: skeletal muscles
    iii) Smooth muscle system
  d) Cardiovascular system
    i) Function: transport nutrients and O_2 to tissues and remove cellular wastes (e.g., urea and CO_2)
    ii) Organs: heart and blood vessels
  e) Respiratory system
    i) Function: exchange of gases (O_2 and CO_2); maintenance of blood pH and electrolytes
    ii) Organs: oral cavity, nose, nasal cavity, pharynx, larynx, trachea, bronchial tubes within lungs, and alveoli
  f) Urinary system
    i) Function: removal of metabolic wastes from blood; maintenance of blood, pH, and electrolytes
    ii) Organs: kidneys, ureters, urinary bladder, and urethra
  g) Integumentary system
    i) Function: protection, excretion, regulation of body temperature, sensory reception, immunity, synthesis of vitamin D, and blood reservoir
    ii) Organs: skin, hair, nails, sweat glands, and sebaceous glands
  h) Digestive system
    i) Function: breakdown of food into substances that can be absorbed for energy
    ii) Organs: mouth, pharynx, esophagus, stomach, small and large intestines, salivary glands, liver, pancreas, and gallbladder
  i) Nervous system
    i) Function: The general function of the nervous system is to coordinate all body systems. This is accomplished by the transmission of (electrochemical) signals from body parts to the brain and back to the body parts; coordination of body parts; control.
    ii) Organs: brain, spinal cord, and nerves
  j) Endocrine system
    i) Function: to integrate body systems (i.e., maintain homeostasis) in conjunction with the nervous system
    ii) Organs: endocrine glands (hypothalamus, pituitary, pineal gland, thyroid, parathyroids, thymus, adrenals, pancreas, testes, and ovaries) that secrete hormones

k) Reproductive system
    i)   Function: production, maintenance, and transport of gametes; production of sex hormones
    ii)   Organs: Male: testes, epididymis, vas deferens, prostate, seminal vesicle, bulbourethral glands, urethra, penis, and scrotum. Female: ovaries, fallopian tubes, uterus, cervix, vagina, labia, and clitoris
l) Lymphatic system
    i)   Function: to prevent edema (accumulation of excess tissue fluid), transport dietary fat, and help fight infection
    ii)   Organs: primary (bone marrow and thymus); secondary (lymph nodes and spleen)
m) Somatic sensory system
    i)   Function: process sensation and perception

Chemistry

The Chemistry section measures knowledge of principles and concepts of inorganic and elementary organic chemistry. Below is a breakdown of the major points you will need to know for the Chemistry section of the PCAT:

General Chemistry

1) **Basic concepts and tools**
   a) Basic concepts:
      i) Physic property: can be measured/observed without changing the composition or identity of a substance
      ii) Chemical property: must carry out a chemical change in order to observe
      iii) Elements: cannot be separated into simpler substances by chemical means
      iv) Compounds: a substance composed of atoms of two or more elements chemically united in fixed proportions
      v) A substance can exist in the following three states: solid, liquid, and gas.
   b) Basic tools:
      i) SI units: K (temperature, absolute zero = $-273.15°C$), kg (mass), m. (meter), s (time), J (energy), etc.
      ii) Significant figures:
         (1) Addition/subtraction: result must round off to the least precise measurement
         (2) Multiplication/division: result must round off to have the same significant numbers as the measurement having the least significant numbers

2) **Atoms, molecules, and ions**
   a) Atoms: usually made up of electrons, protons, and neutrons
   b) Molecules: an aggregate of at least two atoms held together by chemical forces
   c) Ions and ionic compounds
   d) Percent composition by mass: the percent by mass of each element in a compound
   e) Nomenclature of inorganic compounds: binary and ternary compounds; salts

3) **Chemical equations: reactants → products**
   a) Balanced chemical equations: obey the Law of Conservation of Mass; contain the same number of each kind of atom on each side of the equation
   b) Limiting reagent: the reactant used up first in a reaction
   c) Percent yield (% yield) $= \dfrac{\text{actual yield}}{\text{theoretical yield} \times 100\%}$
   d) Ionic equations: show dissolved ionic compounds in their free ions
      Spectator ions: ions not involved in the overall reaction
      Net ion equations: show only species that actually take part in the reaction

4) The periodic table

a) Classification of elements: metals, nonmetals, and metalloids

b) Atomic radius increases down a column and decreases across a row

c) Metallic character of elements within a group increases down a column

5) Chemical bonds

a) Valence electrons: electrons in the outermost shell

b) Ionic bond: transfer of electrons from one atom to another

c) Covalent bond: sharing electrons between two atoms

d) Electronegativity: the ability of an atom to attract toward itself the electrons in a chemical bond. F is the most electronegative element.

e) VSEPR models can predict the geometry of molecules based on repulsion of electron pairs; examples include linear ($BeCl_2$), trigonal planar (BF_3), tetrahedral (CH_4), trigonal bipyramidal (PCl_5) and Octahedral (SF_6) structures

f) Hybridization of atomic orbitals: the mixing of atomic orbitals in an atom to generate a set of new atomic orbitals

g) Hydrogen bond: a special type of dipole-dipole interaction between the hydrogen atom in a polar bond, such as O–H and N–H. In general, only N, O, and F can form hydrogen bonding.

6) The gaseous state of matter

a) Graham's law of gas diffusion or effusion: the diffusion or effusion rates of gases are inversely proportional to the square roots of their molar masses.

b) Boyle's law: $P_1V_1 = P_2V_2$ at constant n, T; n is the number of moles of gas present.

c) Charlie's law: $V \mu T$ at constant n, P

d) Avogadro's law: $V a n$ at constant P, T

e) Ideal gas law: $PV = nRT$

f) STP: the conditions of $0° C$ and 1 atm. One mole of gas occupies a volume of 22.4 liters at STP.

g) Dalton's law: the total pressure of a mixture of gases is the sum of the pressures that each gas would exert if present alone.

7) Solutions

a) Solute: the substance present in smaller amount. Solvent: the substance present in larger amount.

b) In general: polar or ionic compounds dissolve in polar solvents; nonpolar compounds dissolve in nonpolar solvents (like dissolves like).

c) Henry's law: the solubility of a gas in a liquid is proportional to the pressure of the gas over the solution.

d) Molarity:

M = (moles of solute)/(liter of solution)

For dilution or mixing: $M_1V_1 + M_2V_2 + ... = M_{final}V_{final}$

e) Mass percent concentration:

Mass percent = (g solute). 100/(total weight of solution); ppm is part per million; ppb is part per billion.

  f) Normality:

   N = (equivalents of solute)/(liter of solution)

   For dilution or mixing: $N_1V_1 + N_2V_2 + ... = N_{final}V_{final}$

  g) Molality: m = (moles of solute)/(kg solvent)

  h) Electrolyte: the water solution of this substance can conduct electricity. Nonelectrolyte: the water solution of this substance cannot conduct electricity.

  i) Colligative properties of nonelectrolyte solutions: vapor pressure lowing, boiling pressure elevation, freezing pressure depression, and osmotic pressure

  j) Osmosis: diffusion of water into a higher concentrated solution through a semipermeable membrane. Osmosis pressure depends only on the molality of the solution.

8) Acids and bases

  a) Definitions

   i) Arrhenius acid: substances provide H+ in aqueous solution; Arrhenius base: substances provide OH– in aqueous solution

   ii) Brønsted-Lowry acid: a proton donor; Brønsted-Lowry base: a proton acceptor

   iii) Lewis acid: electron-pair acceptor; Lewis base: electron-pair donor

  b) $K_w = [H^+][OH^-] = 1.01 \times 10^{-14}$ at 25°C

  c) pH = –log[H+]. Acidic solution: pH < 7; neutral solution: pH = 7; basic solution: pH > 7. pH + pOH = 14.

  d) For a solution that contains a weak acid and its salt: pH = pKa + log [base]/[acid]

  e) Acid-base reactions:

   i) strong acid + strong base → neutral solution

   ii) strong acid + weak base → acidic solution

   iii) weak acid + strong base → basic solution

   iv) weak acid + weak base → depends on relative values of Ka and Kb

  f) Buffer solutions: composed of a weak acid or base and its salt.

   i) Can resist small change in pH when small amount of acid or base is added

   ii) Selection of buffer solution: desired pH = pKa of the weak acid

   iii) Buffer range: pH range = pKa ± 1

9) Chemical equilibrium

  a) At equilibrium:

   Forward reaction rate = reverse reaction rate

  b) Equilibrium constant for a reaction:

   aA + bB ← → cC + dD

   Equilibrium constant: Keq= [C]c[D]d/[A]a[B]b

  c) Le Chatelier's principle: if a stress is applied to a system in equilibrium, the system will respond in such a way as to relieve that stress and restore equilibrium under a new set of conditions.

10) Oxidation-reduction

   a) Oxidation number: electrons lost, gained, or unequally shared by an atom

   b) Oxidation: losing electrons $\rightarrow$ oxidation number increases $\rightarrow$ is a reducing agent

   c) Reduction: gaining electrons $\rightarrow$ oxidation number decreases $\rightarrow$ is an oxidizing agent

   d) Balancing oxidation-reduction equation: equalize loss and gain of electrons

11) Quantum chemistry

   a) Heisenberg Uncertainty Principle: it is not possible to know the position and the momentum of a particle simultaneously.

   b) Quantum numbers:

     i) The principle quantum number n: the maximum number of electrons that n can hold is $2n^2$.

     ii) The angular momentum quantum number l can have integer values from 0 to n–1; l = 0 $\rightarrow$ s orbital; l = 1 $\rightarrow$ p orbital

     iii) The magnetic quantum number (ml) can have integer values from –l to +l.

     iv) The electron spin quantum number (ms) can only have values of $-\frac{1}{2}$ and $+\frac{1}{2}$.

   c) Pauli Exclusion Principle: no two electrons in an atom can have the same four quantum numbers.

Organic Chemistry

Basic organic compounds and functional groups:

1) **Hydrocarbons: only contain carbon and hydrogen elements; can be divided into aliphatic hydrocarbons (no benzene group) and aromatic hydrocarbons (contain one or more benzene rings); aliphatic hydrocarbons can be further classified as alkanes, alkenes, and alkynes.**

   a) Alkanes: general formula CnH2n+2

   b) Alkenes: general formula CnH2n

   c) Alkynes: general formula of CnH2n–2

   d) Aromatic hydrocarbons

2) **Alcohols: contain hydroxyl group, –OH; general formula: ROH.**

   a) Classification: primary (1°), secondary (2°), or tertiary (3°) alcohols

   b) Oxidation: primary alcohols oxidize to aldehyde and further oxidize to carboxylic acid; secondary alcohols oxidize to ketones; tertiary alcohols normally cannot be oxidized.

   c) Carbon atoms exist in progressively higher stages of oxidation as follows: Alkanes $\rightarrow$ Alcohols $\rightarrow$ Aldehyde or Ketones $\rightarrow$ Carboxylic acids $\rightarrow$ Carbon dioxide. The carbon atoms in CH_4 and CO_2 represent the two extreme oxidation states of carbon, –4 and +4, respectively.

   d) Dehydration: forms alkenes or ethers

   e) Esterification: react with carboxylic acid to form esters. Alcohols lose –OH group and carboxylic acids lose –H group.

   f) Phenol: compounds having a hydroxyl group attached to an aromatic ring. The parent compound is phenol (C_6H_5OH). Phenol is a weak acid, more acidic than alcohols and water, but less acidic than acetic and carbonic acids.

3) **Ethers: general formula of R–O–R'**

4) **Aldehydes and ketones: functional group is carbonyl group (–CO–). Aldehydes have the general formula of R–CHO. Ketones have the general formula of R–CO–R'.**

   a) The carbon atom of the carbonyl group is *sp*2 hybridized.

   b) Aldehydes can be oxidized to carboxylic acids and give a positive Tollen's test (silver-mirror test), Fehling's test, and Benedict test. Normally, ketones cannot be oxidized and do not give positive tests.

   c) Aldehydes and ketones can be reduced to alcohols.

5) **Carboxylic acids: functional group is the carboxyl group, –COOH; general formula is RCOOH.**

   a) Acid chlorides formation: carboxylic acids react with $SOCl_2$ or PCl_5

   b) Acetic acid can form Dimmer's to reduce its polarity.

   c) Ester formation: carboxylic acids react with alcohols

6) **Esters: General formula for esters is RCOOR': R = H, alkyl, or aryl group; R' = alkyl or aryl group, but *not* a hydrogen; –COOR is the functional group.**

    a) Hydrolysis: splitting of molecules through the addition of water

    b) Acid hydrolysis of esters: ester reacts with water to form an acid and an alcohol; catalyzed by strong acids or by certain enzymes

    c) Alkaline hydrolysis (Saponification): hydrolysis of ester by a strong base to form an alcohol and a salt

7) **Amines: general formula is RNH_2 (primary amine), R_2NH (secondary amine), or R_3N (tertiary amine), where R = alkyl or aryl group; amines are organic bases.**

8) **Amides: general formula is $RCONH_2$, RCONHR, or $RCONR_2$; major reaction is hydrolysis.**

Synthetic organic polymers and natural polymers in living systems

1) **Synthetic organic polymers: often called macromolecules; having high molar mass ranging into thousands and millions of grams**

   a) Addition reactions and condensation reactions are two types of polymerization reactions.

   b) Homopolymers: made from only one type of monomer

   c) Copolymerization: formation of polymer containing two or more different monomers

2) **Carbohydrates: polyhydroxy ketones or substances that yield these compounds when hydrolyzed**

   a) Classification: monosaccharides, disaccharides, and polysaccharides (or oligosaccharides)

   b) Monosaccharide: glucose is the most important. Glucose is a reducing sugar and gives a positive Tollen's test.

   c) Disaccharide: sucrose and lactose are two important disaccharides.

   d) Polysaccharide: starch, cellulose, and glycogen are three important polysaccharides.

3) **Lipids: water insoluble, oily or greasy biochemical compounds that can be extracted from cells by nonpolar solvents**

   a) Examples of lipids: fats, oils, steroids (cholesterol belongs to steroids)

4) **Amino acids, polypeptides, and proteins**

   a) Amino acids: general formula RNH_2COOH

      i) Classification: neutral (same number of amino and carboxyl groups), acidic (more carboxyl groups), and basic (more amino groups)

      ii) Glycine NH_2CH_2COOH is the simplest amino acid.

   b) Peptides: amino acid units joined through amide structures

   c) Proteins

      i) Primary structure: the number, kind, and sequence of amino acid units of the peptide chain or polypeptide chains

      ii) Secondary structure: regular, three-dimensional structure held together by hydrogen bonding between the oxygen of the carbonyl and –NH– group. a-helix and b-sheet are two examples.

      iii) Tertiary structure: refers to the distinctive and characteristic shape of a protein

5) **Nucleic acids: DNA and RNA**

   a) Chargaff's rule: the amount of A, G, C, T must satisfy A = T, C = G, and A + G = C + T.

   b) Under normal conditions, an A is paired with a T and a G is paired with a C.

Reading Comprehension

The Reading Comprehension section measures one's ability to comprehend, analyze, and evaluate reading passages on science-related topics. This section contains ten reading passages. Each of the passages is either short (200–600 words) or long (700–950 words) and is followed by a set of questions that directly relate to the passage. There are usually 4–6 questions for short passages and 8–12 questions for long passages. The passages selected for the actual PCAT come from different content areas, including biology, chemistry, and the physical sciences. The actual test contains both long and short passages, with a total of five or six passages. Below are some key points to remember when preparing to answer reading comprehension questions:

- Reading comprehension is based on your reading skills, including understanding new words, developing speed and rhythm in your reading style, and scanning passages quickly and correlating information.

- The PCAT tests your ability to read, organize, and analyze information.

- Because the information explosion is doubling the amount of available information every two years, you will need to be able to read and comprehend a significant amount of literature in a short time.

- New information refers to information that you have not yet seen and information that you have seen at a glance. For instance, in the *Wall Street Journal*, articles are briefly recapped on the front page. It is important to be able to scan these recaps for recognition of new information.

- Reading ability depends on the complexity and difficulty of the reading.

- You must be able to concentrate on reading passages without trying to memorize information as you read.

- Improve your vocabulary daily. Working on crossword puzzles and keeping a log or diary of new words are two ways to increase vocabulary.

- The level of a reading passage depends on the topic, as well as the vocabulary used, in the passage. Increasing your vocabulary will enhance your reading comprehension as well as your verbal ability.

- Reason as you read! If a passage has long complex sentences, break them down into manageable components that you can absorb and analyze. Understanding short phrases will assist you in reading and comprehending complex passages.

- There are several sources of new information that you should begin reading routinely. You do not have to buy these publications; you can read them in the library or your local bookstore. These include, but are not limited to, the following:

American Journal of Hospital Pharmacy

American Journal of Managed Care

American Pharmacy

Journal of the American Medical Association

Nature

PharmacoEconomics

Science

The New England Journal of Medicine

The Wall Street Journal

Time

USA Today

Local newspapers

- Do not read in haste!

- Read and focus on the topic area as well as on the questions. Do NOT answer the questions based on your knowledge but rather on the information provided in the passage. Although your knowledge may be absolutely correct, the passage may focus on a different approach to the topic.

- You may not agree with the statements in the passage, but remember that you are reading to comprehend what appears in the passage.

Critical Thinking Essay

Many colleges of pharmacy require a formal interview as part of the application process. Part of the interview process includes a written essay given to the applicant during the interview. To prepare students for the essay writing portion of the interview, the PCAT now includes a Critical Thinking Essay.

The Critical Thinking Essay is used to measure one's aptitude in language and composition. Examinees have 30 minutes to write an essay in response to a statement that either expresses an opinion on an issue or presents a problem needing a solution.

Scoring

The Critical Thinking Essay score is assigned on a scale of 1 to 5, with 5 representing the highest score possible. The quality of the scores is assured by supervisors who systematically read selected essays to verify that the scores are consistent with pre-established criteria for each score point. An examinee's Critical Thinking Essay score is reported on the personal Score Report and on each official transcript. Scores are based on the following criteria:

SCORE POINT 5—SUPERIOR

The writer is in command of the conventions of language; makes very few, if any, mistakes in sentence formation, usage, and mechanics. Some evidence is shown of advanced or innovative techniques.

SCORE POINT 4—EFFECTIVE

On the whole, the writer correctly applies the conventions of language, though there are some mistakes in sentence formation, usage, or mechanics. However, none of these errors are serious enough to interfere with the overall flow of the response or with its meaning.

SCORE POINT 3—ADEQUATE

The writer is fairly successful in applying the conventions of language. Several mistakes in sentence formation, usage, or mechanics are present. While the density of these errors may interfere with the overall flow of the response, they do not interfere with its meaning.

SCORE POINT 2—MARGINAL

The writer is marginally successful in applying the conventions of language. Patterns of mistakes in sentence formation, usage, and mechanics significantly detract from the presentation. At times the meaning of the response may be weakened.

SCORE POINT 1—WEAK

The writer's achievement in applying the conventions of language is limited. Frequent and serious mistakes in sentence formation, usage, and mechanics make the response difficult to understand.

Tips for Writing an Essay

1. Organize your thoughts before you begin to write.
2. Always write on a topic that is given.
3. Write a shorter essay that is complete rather than a longer one that is difficult to complete in the limited time available.
4. Follow the rules of standard written English.
5. Illustrate your ideas with examples.
6. Proofread your essay.
7. Prior to taking the PCAT, have someone give you a topic and time yourself.
8. Organize your essay using the "three main points" approach—*Introduction; First Point, Second Point, Third Point*; and *Conclusion*.

PCAT STUDY PLAN

Here are eight general tips that will help you improve your PCAT scores:

1 Get at least 8 hours of sleep the night before, eat a good breakfast the morning of the test, and dress comfortably.

2 Know exactly where you have to go to take the examination and allow plenty of time to get to the test center.

3 Arrive at the testing site at least 30 minutes before the examination.

4 Use the practice/review materials in this book and take the practice examination under test conditions.

5 Be sure to bring at least 6 sharpened #2 pencils with erasers and a small hand pencil sharpener.

6 Bring an accurate watch or small clock (that does not make ticking noises).

7 Be sure to bring your picture identification with you to the testing site.

8 Be sure of your test date and that you have a confirmation for your test time and site.

Time management is important on an examination such as the PCAT. The following is a list of things you can do to manage your time and improve your score on the PCAT:

1 Answer every question on the examination.

2 Familiarize yourself with the question types and directions for each content area.

3 Pace yourself and work within the allotted time given for each content area.

4 When you start a section, answer the questions that you know the answers to first.

5 If you do skip questions, make sure you mark your answers in the correct spaces on the answer sheet.

6 Read over all of the answer choices before choosing your answer.

7 Remember that you can write on the examination book and make notes if you are unsure about a question or if you have not answered a question.

8 Do NOT make any stray marks on the examination answer sheet. If you do, be sure to erase them completely.

9 If you need to change an answer on your answer sheet, be sure to erase the answer completely.

10 Do NOT leave any answer blank. You are not penalized for guessing.

11 You cannot use a calculator on the PCAT. Practice the quantitative ability section without the use of a calculator.

12 Answer all of the practice/review questions and take the practice examination the day before you are scheduled for the PCAT.

SUMMING IT UP

- There are six content areas measured by the PCAT in six separate subtests: Verbal Ability, Quantitative Ability, Biology, Chemistry, Reading Comprehension, and the Critical Thinking Essay.

- Try to take the PCAT at least two to three test dates before the deadline for your completed admission portfolio in case you need to take the examination again before the school(s) admissions deadline.

- There is no passing or failing score for this test. The extent to which test results are used in deciding whether or not a person will be admitted to a college of pharmacy varies from one school to another.

- The Critical Thinking Essay score is assigned on a scale of 1 to 5, with 5 representing the highest score possible. The quality of the scores is assured by supervisors who systematically read selected essays to verify that the scores are consistent with pre-established criteria for each score point. An examinee's Critical Thinking Essay score is reported on the personal Score Report and on each official transcript.

PART II

DIAGNOSING STRENGTHS AND WEAKNESSES

CHAPTER 2   Practice Test 1: Diagnostic

ANSWER SHEET PRACTICE TEST 1: DIAGNOSTIC

Reading Comprehension

1. Ⓐ Ⓑ Ⓒ Ⓓ   11. Ⓐ Ⓑ Ⓒ Ⓓ   21. Ⓐ Ⓑ Ⓒ Ⓓ   31. Ⓐ Ⓑ Ⓒ Ⓓ   41. Ⓐ Ⓑ Ⓒ Ⓓ
2. Ⓐ Ⓑ Ⓒ Ⓓ   12. Ⓐ Ⓑ Ⓒ Ⓓ   22. Ⓐ Ⓑ Ⓒ Ⓓ   32. Ⓐ Ⓑ Ⓒ Ⓓ   42. Ⓐ Ⓑ Ⓒ Ⓓ
3. Ⓐ Ⓑ Ⓒ Ⓓ   13. Ⓐ Ⓑ Ⓒ Ⓓ   23. Ⓐ Ⓑ Ⓒ Ⓓ   33. Ⓐ Ⓑ Ⓒ Ⓓ   43. Ⓐ Ⓑ Ⓒ Ⓓ
4. Ⓐ Ⓑ Ⓒ Ⓓ   14. Ⓐ Ⓑ Ⓒ Ⓓ   24. Ⓐ Ⓑ Ⓒ Ⓓ   34. Ⓐ Ⓑ Ⓒ Ⓓ   44. Ⓐ Ⓑ Ⓒ Ⓓ
5. Ⓐ Ⓑ Ⓒ Ⓓ   15. Ⓐ Ⓑ Ⓒ Ⓓ   25. Ⓐ Ⓑ Ⓒ Ⓓ   35. Ⓐ Ⓑ Ⓒ Ⓓ   45. Ⓐ Ⓑ Ⓒ Ⓓ
6. Ⓐ Ⓑ Ⓒ Ⓓ   16. Ⓐ Ⓑ Ⓒ Ⓓ   26. Ⓐ Ⓑ Ⓒ Ⓓ   36. Ⓐ Ⓑ Ⓒ Ⓓ   46. Ⓐ Ⓑ Ⓒ Ⓓ
7. Ⓐ Ⓑ Ⓒ Ⓓ   17. Ⓐ Ⓑ Ⓒ Ⓓ   27. Ⓐ Ⓑ Ⓒ Ⓓ   37. Ⓐ Ⓑ Ⓒ Ⓓ   47. Ⓐ Ⓑ Ⓒ Ⓓ
8. Ⓐ Ⓑ Ⓒ Ⓓ   18. Ⓐ Ⓑ Ⓒ Ⓓ   28. Ⓐ Ⓑ Ⓒ Ⓓ   38. Ⓐ Ⓑ Ⓒ Ⓓ   48. Ⓐ Ⓑ Ⓒ Ⓓ
9. Ⓐ Ⓑ Ⓒ Ⓓ   19. Ⓐ Ⓑ Ⓒ Ⓓ   29. Ⓐ Ⓑ Ⓒ Ⓓ   39. Ⓐ Ⓑ Ⓒ Ⓓ
10. Ⓐ Ⓑ Ⓒ Ⓓ   20. Ⓐ Ⓑ Ⓒ Ⓓ   30. Ⓐ Ⓑ Ⓒ Ⓓ   40. Ⓐ Ⓑ Ⓒ Ⓓ

Biology

1. Ⓐ Ⓑ Ⓒ Ⓓ   16. Ⓐ Ⓑ Ⓒ Ⓓ   31. Ⓐ Ⓑ Ⓒ Ⓓ   46. Ⓐ Ⓑ Ⓒ Ⓓ   61. Ⓐ Ⓑ Ⓒ Ⓓ
2. Ⓐ Ⓑ Ⓒ Ⓓ   17. Ⓐ Ⓑ Ⓒ Ⓓ   32. Ⓐ Ⓑ Ⓒ Ⓓ   47. Ⓐ Ⓑ Ⓒ Ⓓ   62. Ⓐ Ⓑ Ⓒ Ⓓ
3. Ⓐ Ⓑ Ⓒ Ⓓ   18. Ⓐ Ⓑ Ⓒ Ⓓ   33. Ⓐ Ⓑ Ⓒ Ⓓ   48. Ⓐ Ⓑ Ⓒ Ⓓ   63. Ⓐ Ⓑ Ⓒ Ⓓ
4. Ⓐ Ⓑ Ⓒ Ⓓ   19. Ⓐ Ⓑ Ⓒ Ⓓ   34. Ⓐ Ⓑ Ⓒ Ⓓ   49. Ⓐ Ⓑ Ⓒ Ⓓ   64. Ⓐ Ⓑ Ⓒ Ⓓ
5. Ⓐ Ⓑ Ⓒ Ⓓ   20. Ⓐ Ⓑ Ⓒ Ⓓ   35. Ⓐ Ⓑ Ⓒ Ⓓ   50. Ⓐ Ⓑ Ⓒ Ⓓ   65. Ⓐ Ⓑ Ⓒ Ⓓ
6. Ⓐ Ⓑ Ⓒ Ⓓ   21. Ⓐ Ⓑ Ⓒ Ⓓ   36. Ⓐ Ⓑ Ⓒ Ⓓ   51. Ⓐ Ⓑ Ⓒ Ⓓ   66. Ⓐ Ⓑ Ⓒ Ⓓ
7. Ⓐ Ⓑ Ⓒ Ⓓ   22. Ⓐ Ⓑ Ⓒ Ⓓ   37. Ⓐ Ⓑ Ⓒ Ⓓ   52. Ⓐ Ⓑ Ⓒ Ⓓ   67. Ⓐ Ⓑ Ⓒ Ⓓ
8. Ⓐ Ⓑ Ⓒ Ⓓ   23. Ⓐ Ⓑ Ⓒ Ⓓ   38. Ⓐ Ⓑ Ⓒ Ⓓ   53. Ⓐ Ⓑ Ⓒ Ⓓ   68. Ⓐ Ⓑ Ⓒ Ⓓ
9. Ⓐ Ⓑ Ⓒ Ⓓ   24. Ⓐ Ⓑ Ⓒ Ⓓ   39. Ⓐ Ⓑ Ⓒ Ⓓ   54. Ⓐ Ⓑ Ⓒ Ⓓ   69. Ⓐ Ⓑ Ⓒ Ⓓ
10. Ⓐ Ⓑ Ⓒ Ⓓ   25. Ⓐ Ⓑ Ⓒ Ⓓ   40. Ⓐ Ⓑ Ⓒ Ⓓ   55. Ⓐ Ⓑ Ⓒ Ⓓ   70. Ⓐ Ⓑ Ⓒ Ⓓ
11. Ⓐ Ⓑ Ⓒ Ⓓ   26. Ⓐ Ⓑ Ⓒ Ⓓ   41. Ⓐ Ⓑ Ⓒ Ⓓ   56. Ⓐ Ⓑ Ⓒ Ⓓ   71. Ⓐ Ⓑ Ⓒ Ⓓ
12. Ⓐ Ⓑ Ⓒ Ⓓ   27. Ⓐ Ⓑ Ⓒ Ⓓ   42. Ⓐ Ⓑ Ⓒ Ⓓ   57. Ⓐ Ⓑ Ⓒ Ⓓ   72. Ⓐ Ⓑ Ⓒ Ⓓ
13. Ⓐ Ⓑ Ⓒ Ⓓ   28. Ⓐ Ⓑ Ⓒ Ⓓ   43. Ⓐ Ⓑ Ⓒ Ⓓ   58. Ⓐ Ⓑ Ⓒ Ⓓ   73. Ⓐ Ⓑ Ⓒ Ⓓ
14. Ⓐ Ⓑ Ⓒ Ⓓ   29. Ⓐ Ⓑ Ⓒ Ⓓ   44. Ⓐ Ⓑ Ⓒ Ⓓ   59. Ⓐ Ⓑ Ⓒ Ⓓ   74. Ⓐ Ⓑ Ⓒ Ⓓ
15. Ⓐ Ⓑ Ⓒ Ⓓ   30. Ⓐ Ⓑ Ⓒ Ⓓ   45. Ⓐ Ⓑ Ⓒ Ⓓ   60. Ⓐ Ⓑ Ⓒ Ⓓ   75. Ⓐ Ⓑ Ⓒ Ⓓ

answer sheet

Quantitative Ability

1. Ⓐ Ⓑ Ⓒ Ⓓ	21. Ⓐ Ⓑ Ⓒ Ⓓ	41. Ⓐ Ⓑ Ⓒ Ⓓ	61. Ⓐ Ⓑ Ⓒ Ⓓ	81. Ⓐ Ⓑ Ⓒ Ⓓ
2. Ⓐ Ⓑ Ⓒ Ⓓ	22. Ⓐ Ⓑ Ⓒ Ⓓ	42. Ⓐ Ⓑ Ⓒ Ⓓ	62. Ⓐ Ⓑ Ⓒ Ⓓ	82. Ⓐ Ⓑ Ⓒ Ⓓ
3. Ⓐ Ⓑ Ⓒ Ⓓ	23. Ⓐ Ⓑ Ⓒ Ⓓ	43. Ⓐ Ⓑ Ⓒ Ⓓ	63. Ⓐ Ⓑ Ⓒ Ⓓ	83. Ⓐ Ⓑ Ⓒ Ⓓ
4. Ⓐ Ⓑ Ⓒ Ⓓ	24. Ⓐ Ⓑ Ⓒ Ⓓ	44. Ⓐ Ⓑ Ⓒ Ⓓ	64. Ⓐ Ⓑ Ⓒ Ⓓ	84. Ⓐ Ⓑ Ⓒ Ⓓ
5. Ⓐ Ⓑ Ⓒ Ⓓ	25. Ⓐ Ⓑ Ⓒ Ⓓ	45. Ⓐ Ⓑ Ⓒ Ⓓ	65. Ⓐ Ⓑ Ⓒ Ⓓ	85. Ⓐ Ⓑ Ⓒ Ⓓ
6. Ⓐ Ⓑ Ⓒ Ⓓ	26. Ⓐ Ⓑ Ⓒ Ⓓ	46. Ⓐ Ⓑ Ⓒ Ⓓ	66. Ⓐ Ⓑ Ⓒ Ⓓ	86. Ⓐ Ⓑ Ⓒ Ⓓ
7. Ⓐ Ⓑ Ⓒ Ⓓ	27. Ⓐ Ⓑ Ⓒ Ⓓ	47. Ⓐ Ⓑ Ⓒ Ⓓ	67. Ⓐ Ⓑ Ⓒ Ⓓ	87. Ⓐ Ⓑ Ⓒ Ⓓ
8. Ⓐ Ⓑ Ⓒ Ⓓ	28. Ⓐ Ⓑ Ⓒ Ⓓ	48. Ⓐ Ⓑ Ⓒ Ⓓ	68. Ⓐ Ⓑ Ⓒ Ⓓ	88. Ⓐ Ⓑ Ⓒ Ⓓ
9. Ⓐ Ⓑ Ⓒ Ⓓ	29. Ⓐ Ⓑ Ⓒ Ⓓ	49. Ⓐ Ⓑ Ⓒ Ⓓ	69. Ⓐ Ⓑ Ⓒ Ⓓ	89. Ⓐ Ⓑ Ⓒ Ⓓ
10. Ⓐ Ⓑ Ⓒ Ⓓ	30. Ⓐ Ⓑ Ⓒ Ⓓ	50. Ⓐ Ⓑ Ⓒ Ⓓ	70. Ⓐ Ⓑ Ⓒ Ⓓ	90. Ⓐ Ⓑ Ⓒ Ⓓ
11. Ⓐ Ⓑ Ⓒ Ⓓ	31. Ⓐ Ⓑ Ⓒ Ⓓ	51. Ⓐ Ⓑ Ⓒ Ⓓ	71. Ⓐ Ⓑ Ⓒ Ⓓ	91. Ⓐ Ⓑ Ⓒ Ⓓ
12. Ⓐ Ⓑ Ⓒ Ⓓ	32. Ⓐ Ⓑ Ⓒ Ⓓ	52. Ⓐ Ⓑ Ⓒ Ⓓ	72. Ⓐ Ⓑ Ⓒ Ⓓ	92. Ⓐ Ⓑ Ⓒ Ⓓ
13. Ⓐ Ⓑ Ⓒ Ⓓ	33. Ⓐ Ⓑ Ⓒ Ⓓ	53. Ⓐ Ⓑ Ⓒ Ⓓ	73. Ⓐ Ⓑ Ⓒ Ⓓ	93. Ⓐ Ⓑ Ⓒ Ⓓ
14. Ⓐ Ⓑ Ⓒ Ⓓ	34. Ⓐ Ⓑ Ⓒ Ⓓ	54. Ⓐ Ⓑ Ⓒ Ⓓ	74. Ⓐ Ⓑ Ⓒ Ⓓ	94. Ⓐ Ⓑ Ⓒ Ⓓ
15. Ⓐ Ⓑ Ⓒ Ⓓ	35. Ⓐ Ⓑ Ⓒ Ⓓ	55. Ⓐ Ⓑ Ⓒ Ⓓ	75. Ⓐ Ⓑ Ⓒ Ⓓ	95. Ⓐ Ⓑ Ⓒ Ⓓ
16. Ⓐ Ⓑ Ⓒ Ⓓ	36. Ⓐ Ⓑ Ⓒ Ⓓ	56. Ⓐ Ⓑ Ⓒ Ⓓ	76. Ⓐ Ⓑ Ⓒ Ⓓ	96. Ⓐ Ⓑ Ⓒ Ⓓ
17. Ⓐ Ⓑ Ⓒ Ⓓ	37. Ⓐ Ⓑ Ⓒ Ⓓ	57. Ⓐ Ⓑ Ⓒ Ⓓ	77. Ⓐ Ⓑ Ⓒ Ⓓ	97. Ⓐ Ⓑ Ⓒ Ⓓ
18. Ⓐ Ⓑ Ⓒ Ⓓ	38. Ⓐ Ⓑ Ⓒ Ⓓ	58. Ⓐ Ⓑ Ⓒ Ⓓ	78. Ⓐ Ⓑ Ⓒ Ⓓ	98. Ⓐ Ⓑ Ⓒ Ⓓ
19. Ⓐ Ⓑ Ⓒ Ⓓ	39. Ⓐ Ⓑ Ⓒ Ⓓ	59. Ⓐ Ⓑ Ⓒ Ⓓ	79. Ⓐ Ⓑ Ⓒ Ⓓ	99. Ⓐ Ⓑ Ⓒ Ⓓ
20. Ⓐ Ⓑ Ⓒ Ⓓ	40. Ⓐ Ⓑ Ⓒ Ⓓ	60. Ⓐ Ⓑ Ⓒ Ⓓ	80. Ⓐ Ⓑ Ⓒ Ⓓ	100. Ⓐ Ⓑ Ⓒ Ⓓ

Chemistry

1. Ⓐ Ⓑ Ⓒ Ⓓ   21. Ⓐ Ⓑ Ⓒ Ⓓ   41. Ⓐ Ⓑ Ⓒ Ⓓ   61. Ⓐ Ⓑ Ⓒ Ⓓ   81. Ⓐ Ⓑ Ⓒ Ⓓ

2. Ⓐ Ⓑ Ⓒ Ⓓ   22. Ⓐ Ⓑ Ⓒ Ⓓ   42. Ⓐ Ⓑ Ⓒ Ⓓ   62. Ⓐ Ⓑ Ⓒ Ⓓ   82. Ⓐ Ⓑ Ⓒ Ⓓ

3. Ⓐ Ⓑ Ⓒ Ⓓ   23. Ⓐ Ⓑ Ⓒ Ⓓ   43. Ⓐ Ⓑ Ⓒ Ⓓ   63. Ⓐ Ⓑ Ⓒ Ⓓ   83. Ⓐ Ⓑ Ⓒ Ⓓ

4. Ⓐ Ⓑ Ⓒ Ⓓ   24. Ⓐ Ⓑ Ⓒ Ⓓ   44. Ⓐ Ⓑ Ⓒ Ⓓ   64. Ⓐ Ⓑ Ⓒ Ⓓ   84. Ⓐ Ⓑ Ⓒ Ⓓ

5. Ⓐ Ⓑ Ⓒ Ⓓ   25. Ⓐ Ⓑ Ⓒ Ⓓ   45. Ⓐ Ⓑ Ⓒ Ⓓ   65. Ⓐ Ⓑ Ⓒ Ⓓ   85. Ⓐ Ⓑ Ⓒ Ⓓ

6. Ⓐ Ⓑ Ⓒ Ⓓ   26. Ⓐ Ⓑ Ⓒ Ⓓ   46. Ⓐ Ⓑ Ⓒ Ⓓ   66. Ⓐ Ⓑ Ⓒ Ⓓ   86. Ⓐ Ⓑ Ⓒ Ⓓ

7. Ⓐ Ⓑ Ⓒ Ⓓ   27. Ⓐ Ⓑ Ⓒ Ⓓ   47. Ⓐ Ⓑ Ⓒ Ⓓ   67. Ⓐ Ⓑ Ⓒ Ⓓ   87. Ⓐ Ⓑ Ⓒ Ⓓ

8. Ⓐ Ⓑ Ⓒ Ⓓ   28. Ⓐ Ⓑ Ⓒ Ⓓ   48. Ⓐ Ⓑ Ⓒ Ⓓ   68. Ⓐ Ⓑ Ⓒ Ⓓ   88. Ⓐ Ⓑ Ⓒ Ⓓ

9. Ⓐ Ⓑ Ⓒ Ⓓ   29. Ⓐ Ⓑ Ⓒ Ⓓ   49. Ⓐ Ⓑ Ⓒ Ⓓ   69. Ⓐ Ⓑ Ⓒ Ⓓ   89. Ⓐ Ⓑ Ⓒ Ⓓ

10. Ⓐ Ⓑ Ⓒ Ⓓ   30. Ⓐ Ⓑ Ⓒ Ⓓ   50. Ⓐ Ⓑ Ⓒ Ⓓ   70. Ⓐ Ⓑ Ⓒ Ⓓ   90. Ⓐ Ⓑ Ⓒ Ⓓ

11. Ⓐ Ⓑ Ⓒ Ⓓ   31. Ⓐ Ⓑ Ⓒ Ⓓ   51. Ⓐ Ⓑ Ⓒ Ⓓ   71. Ⓐ Ⓑ Ⓒ Ⓓ   91. Ⓐ Ⓑ Ⓒ Ⓓ

12. Ⓐ Ⓑ Ⓒ Ⓓ   32. Ⓐ Ⓑ Ⓒ Ⓓ   52. Ⓐ Ⓑ Ⓒ Ⓓ   72. Ⓐ Ⓑ Ⓒ Ⓓ   92. Ⓐ Ⓑ Ⓒ Ⓓ

13. Ⓐ Ⓑ Ⓒ Ⓓ   33. Ⓐ Ⓑ Ⓒ Ⓓ   53. Ⓐ Ⓑ Ⓒ Ⓓ   73. Ⓐ Ⓑ Ⓒ Ⓓ   93. Ⓐ Ⓑ Ⓒ Ⓓ

14. Ⓐ Ⓑ Ⓒ Ⓓ   34. Ⓐ Ⓑ Ⓒ Ⓓ   54. Ⓐ Ⓑ Ⓒ Ⓓ   74. Ⓐ Ⓑ Ⓒ Ⓓ   94. Ⓐ Ⓑ Ⓒ Ⓓ

15. Ⓐ Ⓑ Ⓒ Ⓓ   35. Ⓐ Ⓑ Ⓒ Ⓓ   55. Ⓐ Ⓑ Ⓒ Ⓓ   75. Ⓐ Ⓑ Ⓒ Ⓓ   95. Ⓐ Ⓑ Ⓒ Ⓓ

16. Ⓐ Ⓑ Ⓒ Ⓓ   36. Ⓐ Ⓑ Ⓒ Ⓓ   56. Ⓐ Ⓑ Ⓒ Ⓓ   76. Ⓐ Ⓑ Ⓒ Ⓓ   96. Ⓐ Ⓑ Ⓒ Ⓓ

17. Ⓐ Ⓑ Ⓒ Ⓓ   37. Ⓐ Ⓑ Ⓒ Ⓓ   57. Ⓐ Ⓑ Ⓒ Ⓓ   77. Ⓐ Ⓑ Ⓒ Ⓓ   97. Ⓐ Ⓑ Ⓒ Ⓓ

18. Ⓐ Ⓑ Ⓒ Ⓓ   38. Ⓐ Ⓑ Ⓒ Ⓓ   58. Ⓐ Ⓑ Ⓒ Ⓓ   78. Ⓐ Ⓑ Ⓒ Ⓓ   98. Ⓐ Ⓑ Ⓒ Ⓓ

19. Ⓐ Ⓑ Ⓒ Ⓓ   39. Ⓐ Ⓑ Ⓒ Ⓓ   59. Ⓐ Ⓑ Ⓒ Ⓓ   79. Ⓐ Ⓑ Ⓒ Ⓓ   99. Ⓐ Ⓑ Ⓒ Ⓓ

20. Ⓐ Ⓑ Ⓒ Ⓓ   40. Ⓐ Ⓑ Ⓒ Ⓓ   60. Ⓐ Ⓑ Ⓒ Ⓓ   80. Ⓐ Ⓑ Ⓒ Ⓓ   100. Ⓐ Ⓑ Ⓒ Ⓓ

answer sheet

Verbal Ability

1. Ⓐ Ⓑ Ⓒ Ⓓ   15. Ⓐ Ⓑ Ⓒ Ⓓ   29. Ⓐ Ⓑ Ⓒ Ⓓ   43. Ⓐ Ⓑ Ⓒ Ⓓ   57. Ⓐ Ⓑ Ⓒ Ⓓ

2. Ⓐ Ⓑ Ⓒ Ⓓ   16. Ⓐ Ⓑ Ⓒ Ⓓ   30. Ⓐ Ⓑ Ⓒ Ⓓ   44. Ⓐ Ⓑ Ⓒ Ⓓ   58. Ⓐ Ⓑ Ⓒ Ⓓ

3. Ⓐ Ⓑ Ⓒ Ⓓ   17. Ⓐ Ⓑ Ⓒ Ⓓ   31. Ⓐ Ⓑ Ⓒ Ⓓ   45. Ⓐ Ⓑ Ⓒ Ⓓ   59. Ⓐ Ⓑ Ⓒ Ⓓ

4. Ⓐ Ⓑ Ⓒ Ⓓ   18. Ⓐ Ⓑ Ⓒ Ⓓ   32. Ⓐ Ⓑ Ⓒ Ⓓ   46. Ⓐ Ⓑ Ⓒ Ⓓ   60. Ⓐ Ⓑ Ⓒ Ⓓ

5. Ⓐ Ⓑ Ⓒ Ⓓ   19. Ⓐ Ⓑ Ⓒ Ⓓ   33. Ⓐ Ⓑ Ⓒ Ⓓ   47. Ⓐ Ⓑ Ⓒ Ⓓ   61. Ⓐ Ⓑ Ⓒ Ⓓ

6. Ⓐ Ⓑ Ⓒ Ⓓ   20. Ⓐ Ⓑ Ⓒ Ⓓ   34. Ⓐ Ⓑ Ⓒ Ⓓ   48. Ⓐ Ⓑ Ⓒ Ⓓ   62. Ⓐ Ⓑ Ⓒ Ⓓ

7. Ⓐ Ⓑ Ⓒ Ⓓ   21. Ⓐ Ⓑ Ⓒ Ⓓ   35. Ⓐ Ⓑ Ⓒ Ⓓ   49. Ⓐ Ⓑ Ⓒ Ⓓ   63. Ⓐ Ⓑ Ⓒ Ⓓ

8. Ⓐ Ⓑ Ⓒ Ⓓ   22. Ⓐ Ⓑ Ⓒ Ⓓ   36. Ⓐ Ⓑ Ⓒ Ⓓ   50. Ⓐ Ⓑ Ⓒ Ⓓ   64. Ⓐ Ⓑ Ⓒ Ⓓ

9. Ⓐ Ⓑ Ⓒ Ⓓ   23. Ⓐ Ⓑ Ⓒ Ⓓ   37. Ⓐ Ⓑ Ⓒ Ⓓ   51. Ⓐ Ⓑ Ⓒ Ⓓ   65. Ⓐ Ⓑ Ⓒ Ⓓ

10. Ⓐ Ⓑ Ⓒ Ⓓ   24. Ⓐ Ⓑ Ⓒ Ⓓ   38. Ⓐ Ⓑ Ⓒ Ⓓ   52. Ⓐ Ⓑ Ⓒ Ⓓ   66. Ⓐ Ⓑ Ⓒ Ⓓ

11. Ⓐ Ⓑ Ⓒ Ⓓ   25. Ⓐ Ⓑ Ⓒ Ⓓ   39. Ⓐ Ⓑ Ⓒ Ⓓ   53. Ⓐ Ⓑ Ⓒ Ⓓ   67. Ⓐ Ⓑ Ⓒ Ⓓ

12. Ⓐ Ⓑ Ⓒ Ⓓ   26. Ⓐ Ⓑ Ⓒ Ⓓ   40. Ⓐ Ⓑ Ⓒ Ⓓ   54. Ⓐ Ⓑ Ⓒ Ⓓ   68. Ⓐ Ⓑ Ⓒ Ⓓ

13. Ⓐ Ⓑ Ⓒ Ⓓ   27. Ⓐ Ⓑ Ⓒ Ⓓ   41. Ⓐ Ⓑ Ⓒ Ⓓ   55. Ⓐ Ⓑ Ⓒ Ⓓ   69. Ⓐ Ⓑ Ⓒ Ⓓ

14. Ⓐ Ⓑ Ⓒ Ⓓ   28. Ⓐ Ⓑ Ⓒ Ⓓ   42. Ⓐ Ⓑ Ⓒ Ⓓ   56. Ⓐ Ⓑ Ⓒ Ⓓ   70. Ⓐ Ⓑ Ⓒ Ⓓ

Critical Thinking Essay

Practice Test 1: Diagnostic

Before you begin to prepare for the PCAT, it's important to know your strengths and the areas where you need improvement. If you find reading comprehension questions easy, for example, it would be a mistake to dedicate hours practicing them. Taking the Diagnostic Test in this chapter will help you determine how you should apportion your study time. Note that the order in which the sections are arranged and the number of questions in this Diagnostic Test may not be the same as the actual exam.

An answer key and explanations follow the test. Do not look at the answers until you have completed the entire Diagnostic Test.

READING COMPREHENSION

48 Questions • 50 Minutes

Directions: Read each of the following passages and choose the one best answer to the questions that follow each passage.

Before the intravenous administration of a medication, it is essential to check the medication, dose, fluid in which the drug is to be given, and time of adminis-
(5) tration against the patient's chart. After this, all the necessary equipment, such as an alcohol or iodophor sponge, a needle, an intravenous board, tape, and the intravenous solution or admixture,
(10) should be assembled. The patient should then be identified by his armband and the procedure explained to the patient to alleviate any apprehension. Venipuncture can then be performed using a needle
(15) or catheter that should be checked after insertion to ensure that it is properly placed in the vein and adequately secured to the patient's arm. The patient should be advised not to disturb the
(20) venipuncture site. Because the rate of flow of the solution can be affected by numerous variables (gravity, solution viscosity, temperature, and possibly defective equipment), it should be checked
(25) every hour or so, depending on hospital policy. When the rate of flow is critical, such as in pediatric patients or in parenteral nutrition, an infusion pump may be needed to ensure the proper flow
(30) of solution into the patient.

1. Which of the following items is NOT part of the necessary equipment for administering an intravenous medication?

    (A) Alcohol sponge or swab

    (B) Needle

    (C) Intravenous solution

    (D) Intramuscular solution

2. Which of the following is a variable that affects the rate of flow of medication?

    (A) Solution color

    (B) Solution viscosity

    (C) Solution smell

    (D) Solution particle size

3. On what kinds of patients should an infusion pump be used?

    (A) Pediatric patients

    (B) Adult patients

    (C) Geriatric patients

    (D) Comatose patients

4. Before administering an intravenous solution, one must check the

    (A) time.

    (B) medication against the chart.

    (C) day.

    (D) dose of the intramuscular drug.

5. After administering an intravenous solution, the rate of flow should be checked

    (A) every hour.

    (B) every half hour.

    (C) periodically.

    (D) per the time specified by hospital policy.

QUESTIONS 6–10 ARE BASED ON THE FOLLOWING PASSAGE.

Adrenergic agents, commonly found in appetite suppressants, bronchodilators, central nervous system stimulants, and vasoconstrictors, produce slight pupil-
(5)   lary dilation. They have not been ob-served to produce any adverse effects in open-angle glaucoma, and the incidence of deleterious effects on angle closure glaucoma after systemic administration
(10) has been extremely low. Adrenergic agents such as epinephrine and phe-nylephrine have been used ocularly to treat open-angle glaucoma. It is impor-tant to note, however, that these agents
(15) will elevate the intraocular pressure by narrowing the anterior chamber angle when instilled into eyes of angle closure patients.
General anesthetics producing para-
(20) sympathetic and sympathetic imbalance may cause pupillary block. To prevent this complication, topical pilocarpine at 1% may be instilled into the eye 1 hour prior to anesthesia.

6. Adrenergic agents are commonly found in all of the following EXCEPT

   (A) bronchodilators.

   (B) bronchoconstrictors.

   (C) vasoconstrictors.

   (D) appetite suppressants.

7. General anesthetics that produce para-sympathetic and sympathetic imbalance may cause pupillary

   (A) constriction.

   (B) dilation.

   (C) block.

   (D) stimulation.

8. Adrenergic agents may cause _____ in intraocular pressure.

   (A) a decrease

   (B) an increase

   (C) a slight change

   (D) no change

9. Which adrenergic agents have been used to treat open-angle glaucoma?

   (A) Epinephrine and ACTH

   (B) Epinephrine and propranolol

   (C) Epinephrine and phenylephrine

   (D) Epinephrine and droperidol

10. Pilocarpine administered _____ hour(s) before anesthesia can prevent the pupil-lary block caused by anesthetics.

   (A) 4

   (B) 2

   (C) $1\frac{1}{2}$

   (D) 1

QUESTIONS 11–15 ARE BASED ON THE FOLLOWING PASSAGE.

There are numerous methods of administering diphenylhydantoin; however, the regimen must be prescribed individually for each patient because of the
(5) many variables that influence the absorption, distribution, metabolism, and excretion of diphenylhydantoin. Ventricular tachycardia usually requires intravenous therapy. There appears to
(10) be no indication in this situation for intramuscular injections, because the drug is slowly and erratically absorbed from the site, besides being very painful. Diphenylhydantoin plasma levels after
(15) intramuscular injection may be 25–50% lower than after equivalent oral doses. Doses of 50–100 mg of diphenylhydantoin, up to a maximum of 1.0 g, may be administered intravenously every 5 min-
(20) utes, producing only a mild decrease (10–30 mmHg) in systolic blood pressure. Single intravenous doses of 300 mg or more produce a more marked hypotension (20–45 mmHg) and also lead
(25) to subtherapeutic diphenylhydantoin plasma levels within 20–40 minutes. Generally, cardiovascular complications can be avoided with an infusion rate of 20–50 mg/min.

11. Treatment of ventricular tachycardia with diphenylhydantoin usually requires

   (A) sublingual therapy.

   (B) intramuscular therapy.

   (C) intravenous therapy.

   (D) subcutaneous therapy.

12. The dose of diphenylhydantoin that may be given intravenously is

   (A) 50–70 mg.

   (B) 50–80 mg.

   (C) 50–100 mg.

   (D) 50–120 mg.

13. With which infusion rate can you avoid cardiovascular complications?

   (A) 20–50 mg/min.

   (B) 20–40 mg/min.

   (C) 20–30 mg/min.

   (D) 10–50 mg/min.

14. At what dose would you expect to see a marked hypotensive effect from diphenylhydantoin?

   (A) 100 mg

   (B) 200 mg

   (C) 250 mg

   (D) 300 mg

15. Which of the following is a reason for NOT administering diphenylhydantoin intramuscularly?

   (A) The procedure is too expensive.

   (B) The drug is erratically absorbed at the site.

   (C) The drug is not absorbed at the site.

   (D) The drug is too unstable.

QUESTIONS 16–20 ARE BASED ON THE FOLLOWING PASSAGE.

In open-angle glaucoma, a physical block-age occurs within the trabecular mesh-work that retards elimination of aque-ous humor. The obstruction is presumed
(5) to be located between the trabecular sheet and the episcleral veins, into which the aqueous humor ultimately flows. The impairment of aqueous drainage elevates the intraocular pressure (IOP)
(10) to 25–35 mmHg (normal, 10–20 mmHg), indicating that the obstruction is usu-ally partial. This increase in IOP is suf-ficient to cause progressive cupping of the optic disk and eventual visual field
(15) defects. As the trabecular spaces be-come more involved, detachment of the cornea and formation of bullae may de-velop. In addition, scotomata (blind spots) may develop. Since visual acuity remains
(20) largely unaffected until late in the dis-ease, presence of scotomata must be re-garded as a major indication for the institution of medical therapy.

16. Open-angle glaucoma is caused by

   (A) physical blockage.

   (B) genetics.

   (C) physical drainage.

   (D) infection.

17. Normal IOP has a range of

   (A) 10–15 mmHg.

   (B) 10–25 mmHg.

   (C) 10–20 mmHg.

   (D) 10–30 mmHg.

18. Increases in IOP may cause all of the following EXCEPT

   (A) progressive cupping of the optic disk.

   (B) visual field defects (over time).

   (C) immediate changes in visual field.

   (D) development of scotomas.

19. Impairment of aqueous drainage elevates the IOP to

   (A) 25–30 mmHg.

   (B) 25–35 mmHg.

   (C) 25–40 mmHg.

   (D) 25–45 mmHg.

20. The obstruction in open-angle glaucoma is presumed to be located between the

   (A) cornea and the iris.

   (B) trabecular sheet and the episcleral veins.

   (C) trabecular sheet and the cornea.

   (D) episcleral veins and the cornea.

QUESTIONS 21–25 ARE BASED ON THE FOLLOWING PASSAGE.

An unusual reaction to quinidine is syncope. Besides loss of consciousness, these syncopal attacks involve pallor, muscular twitching, and sometimes seizures.
(5) When an EKG is obtained during an attack, the pattern indicates ventricular tachyarrhythmia that apparently critically decreases cerebral perfusion, causing loss of consciousness. The attacks
(10) usually terminate spontaneously, but the rare cases of sudden death attributed to quinidine are thought to be secondary to ventricular arrhythmia. On the other hand, this condition is often
(15) observed in patients with coronary artery disease, where sudden death has been reported to occur as a result of the primary cardiac pathological condition rather than from the drug itself. Syn-
(20) cope may occur at low doses (e.g., 0.8 g/day) and without evidence of allergic reactions. An adverse dose-related effect is hypotension, which may occur by alpha-adrenergic receptor blockade or
(25) by a direct negative inotropic effect on the heart.

21. Which of the following is NOT associated with syncopal attacks?

(A) Pallor

(B) Muscular twitching

(C) Loss of consciousness

(D) Itching

22. An adverse dose-related effect of quinidine is

(A) hypertension.

(B) hypotension.

(C) an inotropic effect.

(D) diabetes.

23. When an EKG is obtained during an attack, the pattern indicates

(A) arrhythmia.

(B) ventricular tachyarrhythmia.

(C) ventricular flutter.

(D) atrial tachyarrhythmia.

24. An unusual reaction to quinidine is

(A) ataxia.

(B) pallor.

(C) syncope.

(D) hypotension.

25. Syncope may occur at

(A) high doses of quinidine.

(B) moderate doses of quinidine.

(C) low doses of quinidine.

(D) very high doses of quinidine.

QUESTIONS 26–30 ARE BASED ON THE FOLLOWING PASSAGE.

Many reports have indicated that the tricyclic antidepressants, especially imipramine, may be of benefit in the treatment of MBD in children. However, al-
(5) though most studies have indicated their superiority over placebos, they are still not as effective as the psychostimulants. Further drawbacks associated with their use include the development of toler-
(10) ance in some children and numerous deleterious side effects. Side effects may be somewhat limited by the maximum daily dose approved by the FDA (5 mg/kg per day), but the patient must be
(15) regularly examined for autonomic effects, weight loss, gastrointestinal irritation, fine tremors, hyperirritability, and mood alterations. In addition, the patient should be monitored for more
(20) severe effects on the central nervous system, for example, seizures, and the cardiovascular system, but these can usually be avoided if the practitioner adheres to FDA recommendations. Al-
(25) though the tricyclic antidepressants are helpful in the treatment of MBD in children, their use at this point is experimental and must be accompanied by certain precautions.

26. Which of the following tricyclic antidepressants has been reported to be effective with MBD?

(A) Desipramine

(B) Imipramine

(C) Amitriptyline

(D) Doxepin

27. The maximum daily dose of tricyclic antipressants approved by the FDA is

(A) 5 mg/kg per day.

(B) 10 mg/kg per day.

(C) 15 mg/kg per day.

(D) 20 mg/kg per day.

28. Although the tricyclic antidepressants are superior to placebos, they are still not as effective as

(A) hypnotics.

(B) sedatives.

(C) psychostimulants.

(D) stimulants.

29. The patient must be monitored for more severe side effects on the central nervous system such as

(A) dizziness.

(B) seizures.

(C) headaches.

(D) blindness.

30. Another drawback associated with the use of the tricyclics is

(A) the development of addiction.

(B) sedation.

(C) the development of physical addiction.

(D) the development of tolerance.

QUESTIONS 31–35 ARE BASED ON THE FOLLOWING PASSAGE.

The primary agents in the treatment of MBD are the centrally acting sympathomimetics, for example, methylphenidate, dextroamphetamine, and magnesium
(5) pemoline. This therapeutic approach was first used in 1937, but actual definition and characterization of this indication in pediatric psychopharmacology did not become popular until the late 1960s.
(10) Dextroamphetamine was initially used in 1937 and continued to be the agent of choice until the late 1960s, when methylphenidate usage increased in association with reports of a lower incidence of
(15) side effects with the latter drug. It would appear that these reports of the greater safety of methylphenidate therapy are of questionable clinical significance. Studies attesting to the greater clinical
(20) efficacy of methylphenidate over dextroamphetamine have also been carried out by some authorities who prefer the use of the former drug, while proponents of dextroamphetamine indicate that, in
(25) their hands, it has comparable clinical efficacy at a lower cost.

31. The agent of choice in the treatment of MBD until the late 1960s was

(A) amitriptyline.

(B) dextroamphetamine.

(C) methylphenidate.

(D) magnesium pemoline.

32. Which of the following involves the lowest cost in the treatment of MBD?

(A) Dextroamphetamine

(B) Methylphenidate

(C) Amitriptyline

(D) None of the above

33. Which of the following is NOT a primary agent in the treatment of MBD?

(A) Methylphenidate

(B) Magnesium pemoline

(C) Dextroamphetamine

(D) Chlorpromazine

34. Methylphenidate use increased in the late 1960s due to reports of its

(A) lower cost.

(B) decreased risk of addiction.

(C) lower incidence of side effects.

(D) shorter half-life.

35. The reports of the greater safety of methylphenidate therapy are

(A) conclusive.

(B) still in progress.

(C) of questionable significance.

(D) accepted by all.

QUESTIONS 36–40 ARE BASED ON THE FOLLOWING PASSAGE.

Procainamide may be considered as an alternative to quinidine in the treatment and prophylaxis of atrial fibrillation. Most patients absorb 75–95% of an
(5) oral dose; however, Koch-Weser estimated that 10% of subjects may absorb 50% or less. The uncertainty concerning the dose absorbed and the lag time for stomach emptying into the small bowel,
(10) where the drug is finally absorbed, force the parenteral administration of procainamide in emergencies. Procainamide may be given intravenously at a rate of 25–50 mg/min.
(15) Giardina et al. have intravenously administered 100 mg, up to a maximum of 1 g, every 5 minutes to treat ventricular arrhythmia. This method will produce a minimally effective serum concentration
(20) in 15 minutes. Therapy never had to be interrupted because of hypotension or conduction disturbances; however, the investigators had excluded myocardial infarction patients, who are most sus-
(25) ceptible to these adverse reactions, from their population.

36. Which of the following drugs may be considered as an alternative to quinidine?

(A) Propranolol

(B) Procainamide

(C) Digoxin

(D) Aspirin

37. The dosage used by Giardina et al. to treat ventricular arrhythmias was

(A) 100 mg intravenously every 5 minutes.

(B) 100 mg intramuscularly every 5 minutes.

(C) 200 mg intravenously every 5 minutes.

(D) 200 mg intramuscularly every 5 minutes.

38. The normal rate of intravenous administration of procainamide is

(A) 25–100 mg/min.

(B) 25–75 mg/min.

(C) 25–125 mg/min.

(D) 25–50 mg/min.

39. Most patients absorb what percentage of an oral dose of procainamide?

(A) 65–75%

(B) 65–95%

(C) 75–95%

(D) 55–75%

40. Koch-Weser estimates that 10% of the patients will absorb

(A) 50% or less.

(B) 60% or less.

(C) 70% or less.

(D) 80% or less.

QUESTIONS 41–45 ARE BASED ON THE FOLLOWING PASSAGE.

Corticosteroid-induced glaucoma is well documented. This form of glaucoma is usually painless and involves no ocular findings or visual field defects. The block-
(5) age produced probably occurs in the trabecular meshwork, severely decreasing the outflow of aqueous humor. Systemically or topically administered corticosteroids further hinder outflow, caus-
(10) ing a corresponding increase in intraocular pressure. After topical therapy, a glaucomatous change occurs in the eye instilled with the drug. This ocular hypertensive effect is usually fully revers-
(15) ible within one month after discontinuation of steroid therapy. The increase in intraocular pressure is approximately 10 mmHg for patients with preglaucomatous anterior chambers and
(20) 5 mmHg for normal persons. In some cases, irreversible eye damage occurs if ocular tension persists for one to two months or longer. In addition, cupping of the optic disk and visual field defects
(25) may develop a few months after topical administration of corticosteroids has begun. Patients undergoing chronic topical steroid therapy should therefore have a tonometric examination every two
(30) months.

41. The increase in intraocular pressure is approximately at what level for patients with preglaucomatous anterior chambers?

   (A) 5 mmHg
   (B) 10 mmHg
   (C) 15 mmHg
   (D) 20 mmHg

42. The ocular hypertensive effect caused by corticosteroids is usually

   (A) irreversible.
   (B) fully reversible.
   (C) not seen.
   (D) partially reversible.

43. Irreversible eye damage may occur if ocular hypertension persists for

   (A) two to four months.
   (B) one to two months.
   (C) one to four months.
   (D) two to six months.

44. Corticosteroid-induced glaucoma usually does not involve any of the following symptoms EXCEPT

   (A) pain.
   (B) physical findings in the eye.
   (C) cupping of the optic disk.
   (D) night blindness.

45. Patients undergoing chronic topical corticosteroid therapy should have a tonometric every

   (A) month.
   (B) two months.
   (C) three months.
   (D) four months.

QUESTIONS 46–48 ARE BASED ON THE FOLLOWING PASSAGE.

Art, like words, is a form of communication. Words, spoken and written, render accessible to humans of the latest generations all the knowledge discovered by
(5) the experience and reflection, both of preceding generations and of the best and foremost minds of their own times. Art renders accessible to people of the latest generations all the feelings expe
(10) rienced by their predecessors, and those already felt by their best and foremost contemporaries. Just as the evolution of knowledge proceeds by dislodging and replacing that which is mistaken, so too
(15) the evolution of feelings proceeds through art. Feelings less kind and less necessary for the well-being of humankind are replaced by others kinder and more essential to that end. This is the purpose
(20) of art, and the more art fulfills that purpose, the better the art; the less it fulfills it, the worse the art.

46. The author develops the passage primarily by
    (A) theory and refutation.
    (B) example and generalization.
    (C) comparison and contrast.
    (D) question and answer.

47. According to the author, knowledge is
    (A) evolutionary and emotional.
    (B) cumulative and progressive.
    (C) static and unmoving.
    (D) dynamic and cyclical.

48. According to the passage, all of the following are true EXCEPT:
    (A) Art is a form of communication.
    (B) Art helps to refine sensibilities.
    (C) Art is a repository of experience.
    (D) Real art can never be bad.

BIOLOGY

75 Questions • 45 Minutes

Directions: Choose the one best answer to each of the following questions.

1. The smallest unit of life is the
   - (A) organ.
   - (B) organelle.
   - (C) cell.
   - (D) gene.

2. The organelle primarily responsible for energy production in an aerobic cell is the
   - (A) nucleus.
   - (B) mitochondria.
   - (C) endoplasmic reticulum.
   - (D) Golgi apparatus.

3. In humans, brown eyes (B) are dominant over blue eyes (b). In a cross between two Bb individuals, what percentage of offspring will have blue eyes?
   - (A) 0 percent
   - (B) 25 percent
   - (C) 75 percent
   - (D) 100 percent

4. Solutions that cause red blood cells to shrink are called
   - (A) isotonic.
   - (B) iso-osmotic.
   - (C) hypertonic.
   - (D) hypotonic.

5. A trace element necessary for normal health of the human body is
   - (A) sodium.
   - (B) potassium.
   - (C) calcium.
   - (D) copper.

6. Brown is the dominant color for rats, whereas white is the alternative recessive color. When a homozygous brown rat is crossed with a homozygous white rat, what percentage of the offspring is expected to be brown heterozygous?
   - (A) 25 percent
   - (B) 50 percent
   - (C) 75 percent
   - (D) 100 percent

7. Fat-soluble vitamins include all of the following EXCEPT vitamin
   - (A) A.
   - (B) B.
   - (C) D.
   - (D) K.

8. Under basal conditions, the region of the body that receives the greatest blood flow is the
   - (A) liver.
   - (B) brain.
   - (C) bone.
   - (D) skeletal muscle.

9. Which of the following electrolytes is most abundant in human extracellular fluid?
   - (A) Sodium
   - (B) Potassium
   - (C) Calcium
   - (D) Magnesium

10. Most nutrients are absorbed by which region of the human gastrointestinal tract?

    (A) Stomach

    (B) Colon

    (C) Small intestine

    (D) Large intestine

11. Long-chain fatty acids normally enter the blood system in the form of

    (A) cholesterol esters.

    (B) free fatty acids.

    (C) glycoproteins.

    (D) chylomicrons.

12. The most abundant electrolyte in the intracellular fluid of humans is

    (A) sodium.

    (B) potassium.

    (C) calcium.

    (D) magnesium.

13. In humans, a deficiency in vitamin C (ascorbic acid) is normally associated with

    (A) scurvy.

    (B) rickets.

    (C) pellagra.

    (D) beriberi.

14. Squamous epithelium is normally associated with which region of the human body?

    (A) Kidney

    (B) Lungs

    (C) Skin

    (D) Pancreas

15. Which of the following statements concerning the structure of a cell is false?

    (A) The nucleus of a cell contains DNA and is separated from the surrounding cytoplasm by a nuclear membrane.

    (B) The Golgi apparatus, endoplasmic reticulum, and the majority of chromatin are found in the cytoplasm outside the nucleus.

    (C) A cell with two complete sets of chromosomes is diploid.

    (D) None of the above

16. Which type of muscle will contract most rapidly when stimulated?

    (A) Skeletal

    (B) Cardiac

    (C) Smooth

    (D) All muscle types contract at the same rate.

17. Which statement about fatty acids (triglycerides) is true?

    (A) Most fats containing unsaturated fatty acids are solids at room temperature, whereas fats containing saturated fatty acids are liquids.

    (B) Most fatty acids in nature have an even number of carbon atoms.

    (C) Fats yield approximately 50 percent as much energy as do carbohydrates in humans.

    (D) Saturated fatty acids contain one or more double carbon bonds.

18. The nucleic acid responsible for transmitting genetic information from the DNA molecule in the nucleus to the cytoplasm is

    (A) transfer RNA.

    (B) ribosomal RNA.

    (C) messenger RNA.

    (D) None of the above

19. The proper sequence for the stages of mitosis is

    (A) metaphase, prophase, anaphase, and telophase.

    (B) prophase, anaphase, metaphase, and telophase.

    (C) prophase, metaphase, telophase, and anaphase.

    (D) prophase, metaphase, anaphase, and telophase.

20. Which statement concerning the structure and function of the biological membrane is true?

    (A) Biological membranes are primarily composed of protein with a small layer of lipid on both the inner and outer surfaces.

    (B) Lipid-soluble compounds tend to diffuse through biological membranes faster than water-soluble ones.

    (C) The rate at which lipid-soluble substances pass through biological membranes is determined by the size of the diffusing particle.

    (D) All of the above

21. Passive diffusion of substances through biological membranes

    (A) requires energy sources such as ATP.

    (B) causes a substance to move from a lower to a higher concentration.

    (C) can be inhibited by metabolic poisons such as cyanide.

    (D) is a major process by which uncharged molecules can move through membranes.

22. The ascending (initial) portion of an action potential observed in a cell is caused by

    (A) sodium influx into the cell.

    (B) sodium efflux out of the cell.

    (C) potassium influx into the cell.

    (D) potassium efflux out of the cell.

23. The descending portion of an action potential after the initial spike potential in a cell is caused by

    (A) sodium influx into the cell.

    (B) sodium efflux out of the cell.

    (C) potassium influx into the cell.

    (D) potassium efflux out of the cell.

24. The normal resting potential of the inner side of a nerve cell relative to the outer side is

    (A) 100 mV.

    (B) 50 mV.

    (C) –50 mV.

    (D) –500 mV.

25. Which of the following endogenous substances does NOT actively aid in the digestion of dietary nutrients?

    (A) Pepsin

    (B) Insulin

    (C) Lactase

    (D) Trypsin

26. The organ primarily responsible for detoxifying toxic substances in the blood is the

    (A) lung.

    (B) kidney.

    (C) liver.

    (D) pancreas.

27. In humans, the removal of waste products from the blood is one of the primary functions of the

    (A) liver.

    (B) pancreas.

    (C) kidneys.

    (D) spleen.

28. Absorption of dietary nutrients can be accomplished by which process?

    (A) Active transport
    (B) Facilitated diffusion
    (C) Passive diffusion
    (D) All of the above

29. In humans, bile salts play an important role in enhancing the intestinal absorption of

    (A) fatty acids.
    (B) glucose.
    (C) thiamine.
    (D) amino acids.

30. Which of the following sugars is NOT classified as a simple sugar that can be directly absorbed from the digestive tract in humans?

    (A) Glucose
    (B) Fructose
    (C) Glycogen
    (D) Galactose

31. Which organ of the human body is first affected by a rapid decrease of glucose concentration in the blood?

    (A) Brain
    (B) Heart
    (C) Kidneys
    (D) Eyes

32. In humans, night blindness can be due to a diet deficient in

    (A) iron.
    (B) copper.
    (C) vitamin K.
    (D) vitamin A.

33. The transport process that does not require the presence of a carrier is

    (A) active transport.
    (B) passive diffusion.
    (C) facilitated diffusion.
    (D) None of the above

34. Saturation kinetics are NOT usually observed in which of the following transport processes?

    (A) Active transport
    (B) Passive diffusion
    (C) Facilitated diffusion
    (D) Phagocytosis

35. Which theory states that genes exist in individuals as pairs?

    (A) The theory of recapitulation
    (B) Starling's law
    (C) Mendel's law of segregation
    (D) The Watson-Crick model

36. Of the following, the element least abundant in the human body is

    (A) carbon.
    (B) oxygen.
    (C) hydrogen.
    (D) calcium.

37. Each cell of every organism of a given species contains a characteristic number of chromosomes. How many chromosomes are found in each cell of the human body?

    (A) 13
    (B) 23
    (C) 46
    (D) 48

38. In humans, which blood type is known as the universal donor?

    (A) O negative
    (B) O positive
    (C) AB negative
    (D) AB positive

39. All of the following substances are known to be neurotransmitters at neuromuscular junctions EXCEPT

    (A) epinephrine.

    (B) norepinephrine.

    (C) acetylcholine.

    (D) cholecystokinin.

40. Certain white blood cells are produced in lymphoid tissue such as the spleen, thymus, and lymph nodes. Which of the following white blood cells is produced by lymphoid tissue?

    (A) Neutrophils

    (B) Monocytes

    (C) Eosinophils

    (D) None of the above

41. Immunity produced in response to vaccination with some foreign protein (antigen) is known as

    (A) actively acquired immunity.

    (B) passively acquired immunity.

    (C) natural immunity.

    (D) cellular immunity.

42. The major process by which the kidney removes waste products from the blood is called

    (A) tubular secretion.

    (B) tubular reabsorption.

    (C) glomerular filtration.

    (D) tubular sublimation.

43. Stimulation of the human sympathetic nervous system causes all of the following changes in the body EXCEPT

    (A) increased heart rate.

    (B) increased sweating.

    (C) constriction of pupils.

    (D) increased blood pressure.

44. Fatigue of a muscle that has contracted many times is primarily caused by an accumulation of

    (A) carbon dioxide.

    (B) lactic acid.

    (C) urea.

    (D) sodium chloride.

45. Cell division during which the chromosome number is reduced from diploid to haploid is known as

    (A) mitosis.

    (B) synapsis.

    (C) meiosis.

    (D) karyokinesis.

46. The appearance of any individual with respect to a given inherited trait is known as its

    (A) genotype.

    (B) phenotype.

    (C) recessive trait.

    (D) heterozygous trait.

47. Which of the following disease states is known to be caused by homozygous recessive genes in an individual?

    (A) Sickle-cell anemia

    (B) Beriberi

    (C) Hypertension

    (D) Pellagra

48. Intense exercise and training of an athlete can result in which of the following changes?

    (A) Increase in the number of muscle fibers

    (B) Increased respiratory rate

    (C) Increase in the size of muscle fibers

    (D) A and C

49. During sperm formation, spermatids
    (A) develop directly from primary spermatocytes.
    (B) contain the diploid number of chromosomes.
    (C) develop immediately after the first meiotic division.
    (D) develop immediately after the second meiotic division.

50. An individual with type A negative blood can receive blood from which of the following blood types?
    (A) O negative
    (B) A positive
    (C) O positive
    (D) All of the above

51. Vestigial organs are the remnants of organs that were functional in some ancestral animal. In humans, which organ(s) is NOT vestigial in nature?
    (A) Appendix
    (B) Wisdom teeth
    (C) Coccygeal vertebrae
    (D) Pupils of the eyes

52. Which of the following graphs most accurately shows the relation between the substrate (*S*) and product (*P*) in a saturated irreversible enzymatic reaction?

(A)

(B)

(C)

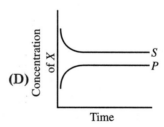

(D)

53. Oxygen and carbon dioxide are primarily transported through the blood
    (A) dissolved in plasma water.
    (B) bound to plasma proteins.
    (C) bound to hemoglobin.
    (D) None of the above

54. Which of the following statements is false concerning the genetics of humans and animals?

   (A) Inbreeding is harmful and leads to the production of genetically inferior offspring.

   (B) Defective traits can be sex linked.

   (C) Outbreeding is the mating of two totally unrelated individuals.

   (D) Vigorous inbreeding can result in a high frequency of defects present at birth, termed congenital anomalies.

55. The members of two different species of animals or plants that share the same living space or food source may interact with each other in a positive or negative manner. Which of the following would be a negative interaction?

   (A) Parasitism

   (B) Commensalism

   (C) Protocooperation

   (D) Mutualism

56. Which of the following graphs most accurately shows the relationship between the substrate (S) and product (P) in a reversible unsaturated enzymatic reaction?

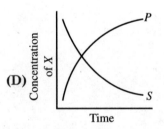

57. Which of the following plasma proteins is most responsible for the osmotic pressure that regulates the water content of the plasma?

   (A) Fibrinogen

   (B) Albumin

   (C) Hemoglobin

   (D) Gammaglobulin

58. Which of the following statements is false concerning leukocytes in the human body?

   (A) Leukocytes are white blood cells.

   (B) Leukocytes move actively by amoeboid movement.

   (C) Leukocytes contain hemoglobin.

   (D) There are the same number of leukocytes as erythrocytes in plasma.

59. Cells that are very important in the production of antibodies for the immune system are

   (A) thrombocytes.

   (B) megakaryocytes.

   (C) neutrophils.

   (D) plasma cells.

60. Which of the following graphs most accurately shows the relationship between the substrate (S) and product (P) in a saturated reversible enzymatic reaction after treatment with cyanide?

(A)

(B)

(C)

(D)

61. The transport of oxygen and carbon dioxide in the blood depends largely on which component of the red blood cell?

   (A) Cell wall

   (B) Nucleus

   (C) Hemoglobin

   (D) Cytoplasm

62. The plasma protein most abundant in plasma is
    (A) albumin.
    (B) globulin.
    (C) fibrinogen.
    (D) immunoglobin.

63. Which of the following conditions does NOT increase the number of red blood cells in the human body?
    (A) High altitude environment
    (B) Low oxygen delivery to the tissues
    (C) Increased erythropoietin production
    (D) Increased carbon dioxide concentration in the blood

64. Which of the following is NOT associated with heat loss in humans?
    (A) Sweating
    (B) Increased muscle tone
    (C) Decreased metabolism
    (D) Vasodilation

65. Substances that are actively reabsorbed by the kidney tubules include
    (A) urea.
    (B) creatinine.
    (C) glucose.
    (D) All of the above

66. Tissues of the body that are normally involved in regulating the volume of body fluids do NOT include
    (A) baroreceptors.
    (B) vasomotor center of the brain.
    (C) osmoreceptor.
    (D) reticular activating system.

67. The structural and functional unit of the nervous system of all multicellular animals is the
    (A) axon.
    (B) nerve.
    (C) neuron.
    (D) dendrite.

68. Which of the following statements about the rate of conduction for a nerve impulse is true in humans?
    (A) The rate of conduction increases as the diameter of the axon increases.
    (B) The rate of conduction is faster in smaller nerve fibers than in larger ones.
    (C) Myelin sheaths usually decrease the rate of conduction.
    (D) All of the above

69. Which of the following statements concerning the human autonomic nervous system is true?
    (A) It controls the voluntary movements of muscles in the limbs.
    (B) It is composed of both sympathetic and parasympathetic nerves.
    (C) Motor impulses reach the effector organ from the brain or spinal cord by a single neuron.
    (D) All of the above

70. In humans, hormones that are derived from amino acids include
    (A) prostaglandins.
    (B) estradiol.
    (C) testosterone.
    (D) thyroxine.

71. When a skeletal muscle fiber is given a single stimulus, a single twitch with numerous electrical phases is observed. What is the correct order for the phases or periods seen in a skeletal muscle fiber after stimulation?

    (A) Contraction, latent, relaxation, refractory
    (B) Refractory, contraction, latent, relaxation
    (C) Latent, contraction, relaxation, refractory
    (D) Latent, refractory, contraction, relaxation

72. Which statement is false concerning the role of hormones in the human body?

    (A) Hormones can be secreted by one part of the body, pass through the blood, and act on a target organ in another part of the body.
    (B) Neurohormones may pass down axons to the target organ in another part of the body.
    (C) Hormones can be derivatives of amino acids, fatty acids, or long peptides.
    (D) Hormones usually provide instantaneous control of a bodily function.

73. Hormones for the regulation of the menstrual cycle in women include

    (A) progesterone.
    (B) vasopressin.
    (C) aldosterone.
    (D) None of the above

74. In the human eye, the rods located in the retina are responsible for

    (A) color vision.
    (B) bright light vision.
    (C) peripheral vision.
    (D) All of the above

75. Which of the following statements is NOT true in reference to the human lymphatic system?

    (A) The rate of lymph flow is similar to that of the circulation.
    (B) The lymphatic system is an auxiliary system for return of fluid from the tissue spaces to the circulation.
    (C) Lymph nodes produce one type of white blood cells, known as lymphocytes.
    (D) The lymphatic system plays an important role in the immune process.

QUANTITATIVE ABILITY

100 Questions • 70 Minutes

Directions: Choose the one best answer to each of the following questions.

1. $\frac{3}{8} + \frac{4}{5} =$
   - (A) $\frac{95}{80}$
   - (B) 1.2
   - (C) $1\frac{7}{40}$
   - (D) $\frac{12}{40}$

2. $0.25 + \frac{15}{16} =$
   - (A) 1.08
   - (B) $1\frac{3}{16}$
   - (C) 3.75
   - (D) $\frac{24}{16}$

3. $1.30 \times 236 =$
   - (A) 3.068×10^2
   - (B) $3,068 \times 10^1$
   - (C) 283.2
   - (D) 29.9×10^2

4. $\log(50 \times 2) =$
   - (A) $(\log 50) \times (\log 2)$
   - (B) $(\log 2) \times (10 \log 5)$
   - (C) $\log 10$
   - (D) $\log 2 + \log 50$

5. $\log 0.001 =$
   - (A) 3
   - (B) 100
   - (C) -3
   - (D) $\frac{1}{3}$

6. $\sqrt[3]{8} =$
   - (A) 2^3
   - (B) $\frac{8}{2}$
   - (C) $8^{\frac{1}{3}}$
   - (D) $8 \log 3$

7. $\log_{10} 1,000 =$
   - (A) 10
   - (B) 3
   - (C) 100
   - (D) 4

8. $1 \times 10^{-2} + 2.3 \times 10^1 =$
   - (A) 2.3×10^2
   - (B) 24.0
   - (C) 23.01
   - (D) 23.1

9. $\frac{3}{16} =$
   - (A) 25%
   - (B) $\frac{9}{32}$
   - (C) 18.75%
   - (D) 33%

10. $\dfrac{(2.3 \text{ g})}{(10 \text{ ml})} =$

 (A) 2.3%

 (B) 0.23%

 (C) 23% $\dfrac{\text{wt}}{\text{vol}}$

 (D) $\dfrac{2.3}{100}$

11. How many liters of a 4% solution can be made from 24 g of a drug?

 (A) 6 liters

 (B) 0.6 liter

 (C) 0.096 liter

 (D) 96 liters

12. How much 0.9% NaCl can be made from 1 liter of an 18% stock solution of NaCl?

 (A) 0.05 liter

 (B) 5.0 liters

 (C) 2.0 liters

 (D) 20 liters

13. What is the percentage of ethanol in a mixture composed of 5 liters of 25%, 2 liters of 50%, and 0.5 liter of 10% ethanol?

 (A) 11.3%

 (B) 50%

 (C) 30.7%

 (D) 22%

14. $\log \sqrt{25} =$

 (A) $\dfrac{1}{2} \log 25$

 (B) $\log 25^{\frac{1}{2}}$

 (C) $\log 5$

 (D) All of the above

15. $\log 25^2 =$

 (A) $\log 50$

 (B) 5

 (C) $\log 5$

 (D) $2 \times \log 25$

16. If 1 kg equals 2.2 lb, how many grams are in 1 lb?

 (A) 454.5 g

 (B) 2,200 g

 (C) 97.8 g

 (D) 1,200 g

17. Subtract 283 ml from 1 liter.

 (A) 217 ml

 (B) 9,717 ml

 (C) 717 ml

 (D) None of the above

18. If 15.43 grains are in 1 g, how many milligrams equals 1 grain?

 (A) 0.065 mg

 (B) 984.6 mg

 (C) 84.57 mg

 (D) 64.81 mg

19. $\sqrt[3]{3^6} + \sqrt{2^2} =$

 (A) 7

 (B) 11

 (C) 36

 (D) None of the above

20. $\left(\dfrac{2}{3}\right)^2 + 2^{-3} =$

 (A) $\dfrac{41}{72}$

 (B) $\dfrac{4}{48}$

 (C) $\dfrac{2}{24}$

 (D) $\dfrac{2}{3}$

21. $10^0 + 10^1 + 10^{-1} =$

 (A) 10.1

 (B) 101

 (C) 11.1

 (D) 1.1

22. If 9 (x°C) = 5(y°F) – 160, what is 79°F in degrees centigrade?

(A) 23.5°C

(B) 87.1°C

(C) 26.1°C

(D) 174.2°C

23. What is –10°C in degrees Fahrenheit?

(A) 50°F

(B) 14°F

(C) –12.2°F

(D) –10°F

24. If the temperature dropped from 72°F to 65°F, by how many degrees centigrade did the temperature change?

(A) 7°C

(B) 13.9°C

(C) 44.6°C

(D) 3.9°C

25. What weight of a particular substance is needed to produce 200 ml of a 1:10,000 solution?

(A) 1 g

(B) 200 mg

(C) 0.02 g

(D) 2 mg

QUESTIONS 26–30 REFER TO THE FOLLOWING GRAPH.

26. At 20 minutes, how much drug remained in the plasma?

(A) 2 mg/ml

(B) There was no change.

(C) 3.5 mg/ml

(D) It cannot be determined.

27. At what rate is the drug disappearing from the plasma?

(A) 2 mg/ml plasma per 60 minutes

(B) 4 mg/ml plasma per 80 minutes

(C) 1.5 mg/ml plasma per hour

(D) None of the above

28. At 2 hours, what would be the concentration of drug in the plasma?

(A) 0.5 mg/ml

(B) 1 mg/ml

(C) No drug will remain.

(D) None of the above

29. If the initial drug concentration had been 8 mg/ml and the rate of disappearance stayed the same, what would have been the drug concentration at 80 minutes?

(A) 6 mg/ml

(B) 4 mg/ml

(C) 2 mg/ml

(D) None of the above

30. How long would it take the drug concentration to reach 0 mg/ml if the initial concentration was 4 mg/ml?

(A) 2 hours

(B) 200 minutes

(C) 160 minutes

(D) 150 minutes

FOR QUESTIONS 31 AND 32, FIND ALL POSITIVE *INTEGERS* SATISFYING THE INEQUALITY.

31. $4 < 3x - 2 \le 10$
    (A) 5, 6, 7, 8, 9, 10
    (B) 1, 2, 3
    (C) 3, 4
    (D) None of the above

32. $\frac{7}{x} > 2$, with $x \ne 0$
    (A) 7
    (B) 1, 2, 3
    (C) 2, 7
    (D) None of the above

33. $|-5| - |-2| =$
    (A) -3
    (B) 7
    (C) 3
    (D) -7

34. $|8| - |14| =$
    (A) 6
    (B) -6
    (C) 22
    (D) None of the above

35. Solve $|5x + 4| = -3$ for x.
    (A) $\frac{7}{5}$
    (B) $\frac{1}{5}$
    (C) 2
    (D) None of the above

QUESTIONS 36–38 REFER TO THE FOLLOWING DIAGRAM.

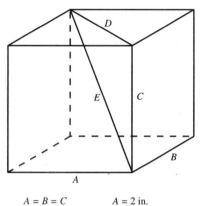

$A = B = C$ $A = 2$ in.

36. What is the length of line D?
    (A) 2 in
    (B) $\sqrt{8}$ in
    (C) 4 in
    (D) $\sqrt{5}$ in

37. What is the area encompassed by lines C, D, and E?
    (A) $\sqrt{8}$ in.^{2}
    (B) $2\sqrt{3}$ in.^{2}
    (C) 2 in.^{2}
    (D) 4 in.^{2}

38. What is the total surface area of the cube?
    (A) 24 in.^{2}
    (B) 16 in.^{2}
    (C) 12 in.^{2}
    (D) 32 in.^{2}

QUESTIONS 39–42 REFER TO THE FOLLOWING DIAGRAM.

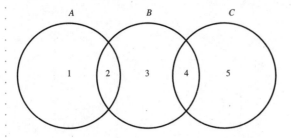

39. The subset A <u>or</u> B encompasses area(s)

(A) 1 and 3

(B) 2 only

(C) 1, 2, and 3

(D) 1, 2, 3, and 4

40. The subset A <u>and</u> B encompasses area(s)

(A) 1 and 3

(B) 2 only

(C) 1, 2, and 3

(D) 1, 2, 3, and 4

41. The subset A or C, <u>but not</u> B, encompasses area(s)

(A) 1 and 5

(B) 1, 2, 4, and 5

(C) 2 and 4

(D) 1, 4, and 5

42. The subset B <u>only</u> encompasses area(s)

(A) 1 and 3

(B) 2, 3, and 4

(C) 2 and 4

(D) 3 only

QUESTIONS 43–45 REFER TO THE FOLLOWING DIAGRAMS.

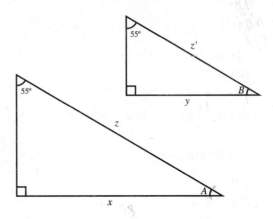

43. If $x = 2y$, what is the ratio of the areas of the two triangles (x:y) above?

(A) 2:1

(B) 4:1

(C) 1:2

(D) $\sqrt{2}$:1

44. How many degrees are there in angle A?

(A) 60°

(B) 45°

(C) 90°

(D) 35°

45. If $x = 3y$ and $z = 5$, what is z'?

(A) $\sqrt{5}$

(B) 3

(C) $\dfrac{3}{5}$

(D) $1\dfrac{2}{3}$

QUESTIONS 46 AND 47 REFER TO THE FOLLOWING GRAPH.

Percentage of drug assayed as compared to the manufacturer's declared amount.

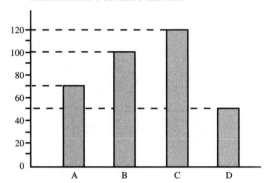

46. If a minimum of 90% of the declared amount of active drug is required by law, which drugs may be used?

(A) C only

(B) B and C

(C) A, B, and C

(D) None of the above

47. If the amount of drug declared by the manufacturer was 200 mg, how much drug was present in the drug samples accepted in the previous question?

(A) 200 mg

(B) 100 and 120 mg

(C) 200 and 240 mg

(D) None of the above

QUESTIONS 48–50 REFER TO THE FOLLOWING GRAPH.

Scores on Final Exam (Percent)

48. What is the mean percent score for the final exam?

(A) 70%

(B) 60%

(C) 66%

(D) 80%

49. What is the modal score?

(A) 70%

(B) 60%

(C) 66%

(D) 80%

50. What is the median score?

(A) 70%

(B) 60%

(C) 66%

(D) 80%

51. If 50 tablets contain 0.625 g of active ingredient, how many tablets can be prepared from 31.25 g of ingredient?

(A) 2,500 tablets

(B) 25 tablets

(C) 625 tablets

(D) 100 tablets

52. The adult (weight 150 lb) dose of a drug is 70 µg. Approximately what is the dose for a child weighing 44 lb?

    (A) 200 µg

    (B) 20 µg

    (C) 3 µg

    (D) None of the above

53. If $x = \frac{1}{y}$, what happens to y when x is increased to $2x$?

    (A) y increases by a factor of 2.

    (B) y decreases by a factor of $\frac{1}{2}$.

    (C) There is no change in y.

    (D) y increases by a factor of 4.

54. If $x = 2y$, what happens to y when x is increased to $2x$?

    (A) y increases by a factor of 2.

    (B) y decreases by a factor of $\frac{1}{2}$.

    (C) There is no change in y.

    (D) y increases by a factor of 4.

55. A quantity of drug weighing 24 g is divided into 16 equal parts. How much does each part weigh?

    (A) 150 mg

    (B) 2,666 mg

    (C) 0.150 g

    (D) 1,500 mg

56. If there may be a 10% error in the weight of a tablet, what is the range of acceptable tablet weights when a tablet of 150 g is desired?

    (A) 135–150 g

    (B) 140–160 g

    (C) 130–170 g

    (D) 135–165 g

57. If there are 65 mg of elemental iron in 325 mg of ferrous sulfate, what percentage of the tablet weight is due to the iron?

    (A) 20%

    (B) 2%

    (C) 5%

    (D) 50%

58. A compound has a maximal solubility of 50 mg/ml. How much is needed to make a 1 liter solution at the maximal concentration?

    (A) 5,000 mg

    (B) 20 g

    (C) 1,000 mg

    (D) 50 g

59. If a graduated cylinder is marked in 5-ml intervals, what is the smallest volume that can be measured with a 10% error?

    (A) 5 ml

    (B) 50 ml

    (C) 100 ml

    (D) 10 ml

60. Give the average of the following to the nearest whole number: 61, 50, 100, 50.

    (A) 50

    (B) 65

    (C) 55

    (D) It cannot be determined.

diagnostic test

QUESTIONS 61–63 REFER TO THE FOLLOWING GRAPH.

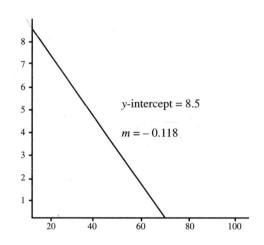

y-intercept = 8.5

$m = -0.118$

61. What is the equation for the line?

(A) $y = 8.5 + 0.118x$

(B) $8.5y = 0.118x$

(C) $y = -0.118x + 8.5$

(D) $y = -\dfrac{0.118x}{8.5}$

62. If y equals 6, what is the value of x to the nearest whole number?

(A) 21

(B) 40

(C) 123

(D) 10

63. If $x = 0$, what is the value of y?

(A) 0.0

(B) 0.118

(C) 8.5

(D) None of the above

QUESTIONS 64–66 REFER TO THE FOLLOWING DIAGRAM.

64. What is the volume of the cylinder ($\pi = 3.14$)?

(A) 987 cubic units

(B) 314 cubic units

(C) 126 cubic units

(D) 63 cubic units

65. What is the lateral surface area of the cylinder?

(A) 987 square units

(B) 314 square units

(C) 126 square units

(D) 63 square units

66. What is the total surface area of the cylinder?

(A) 314 square units

(B) 151 square units

(C) 126 square units

(D) 135 square units

67. What is the area of the trapezoid when $a = 4$, $b = 2$, and $h = 1$?

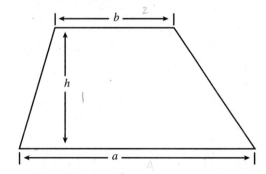

(A) 4 square units

(B) 3 square units

(C) 6 square units

(D) 8 square units

68. What is the area of the parallelogram when $b = 5$ and $h = 2$?

(A) 5 square units

(B) 20 square units

(C) 10 square units

(D) 2.5 square units

69. If $y = 3a + b$ and $x = 3b + a$, find y in terms of x and b.

(A) $3b + 8x$

(B) $3b - 8x$

(C) $3x - 8b$

(D) $3x + 8b$

70. Given the equation $y = mx + c$, a linear plot of y versus x will yield a(n)

(A) slope of m.

(B) ordinate intercept of $\frac{1}{c}$.

(C) abscissa intercept of c.

(D) All of the above

71. $\dfrac{(7 \div 3)}{(21 \div 3)} =$

(A) $\dfrac{7}{21}$

(B) $\dfrac{1}{3}$

(C) 0.33

(D) All of the above

72. Reduce $\dfrac{72}{2,880}$ to lowest terms.

(A) $\dfrac{1}{120}$

(B) $\dfrac{1}{124}$

(C) $\dfrac{1}{52}$

(D) $\dfrac{1}{40}$

73. A prescription calls for 7.5 mg of a drug. How many tablets containing 0.25 mg of the drug are required?

(A) 30

(B) 31

(C) 15

(D) 17

74. Add $\frac{3}{4}$ mg, 0.25 mg, $\frac{2}{5}$ mg, and 2.75 mg.

(A) 5.0 mg

(B) 4.0 mg

(C) 4.15 mg

(D) 5.15 mg

75. Add 0.75 mg, 50 g, and .5 kg.

(A) 550.00075 g

(B) 500.75 g

(C) 0.5575 kg

(D) 500,575 mg

76. $3\frac{1}{8}$ is the same as

(A) $\dfrac{75}{36}$

(B) $\dfrac{100}{32}$

(C) $\dfrac{125}{32}$

(D) $\dfrac{125}{36}$

77. If 60 mg = 1 grain, then 10% of 360 mg =

(A) 6 grain

(B) 0.6 grain

(C) 0.06 grain

(D) 60 grain

78. $2\sqrt{36} + \dfrac{4\sqrt{28}}{3\sqrt{7}} =$

   (A) $14\sqrt{7}$

   (B) $12\dfrac{2}{3}$

   (C) $13\sqrt{7}$

   (D) $14\dfrac{2}{3}$

79. If $A = e^a$, then $1 + A =$

   (A) $1 + e^a$

   (B) e^a

   (C) $\dfrac{1}{e^a}$

   (D) $\ln e^a$

80. $7.7 \times 10^0 =$

   (A) 0

   (B) 0.77

   (C) 7.7

   (D) 77

81. 1,000,000 can also be expressed as

   (A) $1 \times 10^6 \times 10^1$

   (B) $1 \times 10^3 \times 10^{-3}$

   (C) $1 \times 10^3 \times 10^3$

   (D) $1 \times 10^6 \times 10^{-3}$

82. $\sqrt{144 \times 10^4} =$

   (A) 2,400

   (B) 800

   (C) 1,600

   (D) 1,200

83. If 1 kg = 2.2 lb., add the following and express the answer in kilograms: 132 lb., 11 lb., and 44 lb.

   (A) 85 kg

   (B) 88 kg

   (C) 98 kg

   (D) 58 kg

84. $\left(\dfrac{3}{4}\right)^2 + 3^2 + \sqrt{\dfrac{49}{256}} =$

   (A) 27

   (B) 10

   (C) 29

   (D) 30

85. A given line has a slope of –2 and a y-intercept $(0, \sqrt{2})$. It can be expressed as the linear equation

   (A) $y = -2x$

   (B) $y = \sqrt{2} + 2x$

   (C) $y = -2x + \sqrt{2}$

   (D) $y = 2x$

86. Find the value of $\dfrac{250,000 \times 0.018}{0.15}$.

   (A) 300,000

   (B) 275,000

   (C) 37,000

   (D) 30,000

87. What is x if $x^{-3} = \dfrac{1}{27}$?

   (A) 3

   (B) $\dfrac{1}{3}$

   (C) 0.6

   (D) 9

88. What is I ?

   (A) $\dfrac{KH}{J}$

   (B) $\dfrac{JH}{K}$

   (C) $\dfrac{JK}{H}$

   (D) None of the above

QUESTIONS 89–93 REFER TO THE FOLLOWING STATEMENT.

A compound is composed (by weight) of drug A, 20%; drug B, 5%; and drug C, 75%

89. What amount of drug A is required to make 500 g of the compound?

    (A) 100 g

    (B) 125 g

    (C) 375 g

    (D) 400 g

90. What amount of drugs A and B is needed to make 500 g of the compound?

    (A) 100 g

    (B) 125 g

    (C) 375 g

    (D) 400 g

91. What amount of drugs B and C is needed to make 500 g of the compound?

    (A) 100 g

    (B) 125 g

    (C) 375 g

    (D) 400 g

92. What amount of drugs A, B, and C is needed to make 100 g of the compound?

    (A) 100 g

    (B) 125 g

    (C) 375 g

    (D) 400 g

93. What are the ratios A:B:C as indicated in the formula?

    (A) 4:15:1

    (B) 4:1:15

    (C) 15:1:4

    (D) None of the above

94. Given that $\dfrac{B-p}{q} = \dfrac{\frac{g_a}{M_a}}{\frac{g_b}{M_b}}$, find g_b.

    (A) $\left[\dfrac{B-p}{q}\right]\left[\dfrac{M_a M_b}{g_a}\right]$

    (B) $\left[\dfrac{p-B}{q}\right]\left[\dfrac{M_b g_a}{M_a}\right]$

    (C) $\left[\dfrac{q}{B-p}\right]\left[M_b M_a M_a\right]$

    (D) $\left[\dfrac{q}{B-p}\right]\left[\dfrac{M_b g_a}{M_a}\right]$

95. Consider the following:

Equation 1 $y = 3x + 4$

Equation 2 $y = 3x - 4$

Which best describes equations 1 and 2, respectively?

    (A) Slope of +4, y-intercept of +3, slope of −4, and y-intercept of −3

    (B) x-intercept of +3, slope of +4, x-intercept of −3, and slope of −4

    (C) y-intercept of +3, slope of +4, y-intercept of −3, and slope of −4

    (D) Slope of +3, y-intercept of +4, slope of +3, and y-intercept of −4

96. For the following equations, solve for a and b:

$30 = a + 3b - 70$ and $3a + 5b = 100$

    (A) $a = -50, b = 50$

    (B) $a = 5, b = -5$

    (C) $a = -5, b = 5$

    (D) $a = 50, b = -50$

97. How much medicine would provide a patient with 2 tablespoons twice a day for 10 days? (1 tablespoon = 15 ml)

    (A) 300 ml

    (B) 600 ml

    (C) 450 ml

    (D) 900 ml

98. If 0.060 g of a substance is employed in preparing 125 tablets, how much substance is contained in each tablet?

    (A) .390 mg

    (B) .420 mg

    (C) .450 mg

    (D) .480 mg

99. A patient's eye patch measures 12.70 cm across. You have a tape measure in inches. How many inches does the eye patch measure? (1 in. = 2.54 cm)

    (A) 17 in.

    (B) 10 in.

    (C) 5 in.

    (D) 3 in.

100. $\left(\dfrac{1}{120} \div \dfrac{1}{150} \right) \times 50 =$

    (A) $62\dfrac{1}{2}$

    (B) 40

    (C) $50\dfrac{1}{2}$

    (D) 25

CHEMISTRY

100 Questions • 50 Minutes

Directions: Choose the one best answer to each of the following questions.

1. Alkanes are NOT
   (A) saturated compounds containing carbon and hydrogen.
   (B) formed from sp^3 hybrid orbitals.
   (C) arranged in a straight-chain sequence.
   (D) of the general formula C_nH_{2n}.

2. Regarding phenol,
   (A) a nitro substituent in the ortho position will lower the K_a.
   (B) methyl substituent in the ortho position will lower the K_a.
   (C) methyl substituent in the ortho position will increase the K_a.
   (D) the OH substituent is a meta-directing group.

3. Which of the following is true?
   (A) $pH = \dfrac{(\log 1)}{\left[H^+\right]}$
   (B) $pH + pOH = 14$
   (C) $(H+)(OH-) = 10^{-14}$
   (D) $pH - pOH = 14$

4. Calculate the percentage of iron in hematite (Fe_2O_3), given the atomic weights of $Fe = 56$ and $O = 16$.
   (A) 70%
   (B) 2%
   (C) 30%
   (D) 49%

5. How many liters of hydrogen are required to produce 20 liters of ammonia, given the equation $3H_2 + N_2 \rightarrow 2NH_3$?
   (A) 15 liters
   (B) 30 liters
   (C) $33\dfrac{1}{3}$ liters
   (D) 40 liters

6. The volume occupied by the gram-molecular weight of a gas at 0°C and 760 mmHg is
   (A) 1 liter.
   (B) 22.4 liters.
   (C) 32 liters.
   (D) 100 liters.

7. Given the atomic weights of $C = 12$ and $O = 16$, what is the weight of 2 liters of carbon dioxide at standard temperature and pressure?
   (A) 2 g
   (B) 4 g
   (C) 6 g
   (D) 8 g

8. Which of the following hybrid orbitals would carbon form in acetylene?
   (A) sp
   (B) sp^2
   (C) sp^3
   (D) All of the above

9. Which of the following hybrid orbitals would methane and water both form?

    (A) *sp*

    (B) *sp²*

    (C) *sp³*

    (D) All of the above

10. The structural formula indicates all of the following EXCEPT the

    (A) number of atoms in a molecule.

    (B) gram-molecular volume.

    (C) types of atoms present.

    (D) arrangement of the atom.

11. Pick out the incorrect statement.

    (A) Organic compounds may exist as isomers.

    (B) Reactions involving organic compounds always proceed faster than those involving inorganic compounds.

    (C) Organic compounds are generally soluble in organic solvents.

    (D) Organic compounds decompose at relatively lower temperatures than inorganic compounds.

12. When the nucleus of an atom emits a beta particle, the atomic

    (A) weight decreases by 4.

    (B) weight increases by 1.

    (C) number increases by 1.

    (D) number stays the same.

13. The conversion of one element into another is termed

    (A) transformation.

    (B) disintegration.

    (C) transmutation.

    (D) emanation.

14. All of the following are characteristics of gamma rays EXCEPT

    (A) high-energy X rays.

    (B) very short wavelength.

    (C) deflected by electric fields.

    (D) travel at the speed of light.

15. The energy released in nuclear reactions is due to

    (A) atomic fusion.

    (B) electron capture.

    (C) atomic fission.

    (D) both fusion and fission.

16. All of the following are alcohols EXCEPT

    (A) methanol.

    (B) ethanol.

    (C) glycerine.

    (D) sodium hydroxide.

17. Pick out the incorrect statement concerning hydrogen chloride gas.

    (A) It is lighter than air.

    (B) It has a pungent smell.

    (C) It is soluble in water.

    (D) It reacts with ammonia-forming ammonium chloride.

18. All of the following are halogens EXCEPT

    (A) bromine.

    (B) iodine.

    (C) chlorine.

    (D) turpentine.

19. The number of equivalents per mole for $HC_2H_3O_2$ is

    (A) 1

    (B) 2

    (C) 3

    (D) 4

20. Avogadro's law states that
    (A) under identical temperature and pressure, only certain gases contain the same number of molecules.
    (B) all gases contain different numbers of molecules, irrespective of pressure or temperature conditions.
    (C) only under equal volumes will all gases contain the same number of molecules.
    (D) under identical conditions of temperature and pressure, equal volumes of all gases contain the same number of molecules.

21. There are how many different configurations for 2-chlorobutane?
    (A) 8
    (B) 1
    (C) 2
    (D) 6

22. The absolute configuration of a chiral molecule may be assigned using the symbols
    (A) cis and trans.
    (B) R and S.
    (C) syn and anti.
    (D) alpha and beta.

23. Calculate the amount of sodium chloride crystals needed to supply 100 mg of sodium ions (Na = 23, Cl = 35.5).
    (A) 180 mg
    (B) 432 mg
    (C) 355 mg
    (D) 254 mg

24. Calculate the concentration (in milligrams per milliliter) of a solution containing 2 mEq of sodium chloride per milliliter.
    (A) 585 mg/ml
    (B) 355 mg/ml
    (C) 230 mg/ml
    (D) 117 mg/ml

25. It has been ordered that Mr. Smith should receive 2 mEq of sodium chloride per kilogram of body weight. Since Mr. Smith weighs 60 kg, how much sodium chloride is needed?
    (A) 7 g
    (B) 17 g
    (C) 27 g
    (D) 117 g

26. Since the hospital stocks a 0.9% solution of sodium chloride, how much of this solution must be administered to Mr. Smith?
    (A) 777 ml
    (B) 350 ml
    (C) 3,500 ml
    (D) 7,700 ml

27. The pharmacy, however, could only supply a 0.45% solution of sodium chloride. How many liters of this solution must be given to Mr. Smith?
    (A) 1.5 liters
    (B) 3.0 liters
    (C) 4.5 liters
    (D) 6.0 liters

28. Electrolytes (e.g., sodium chloride) are important in establishing osmotic pressure; the unit used in measuring osmotic activity is the milliosmol. How many milliosmols of particles does 1 mole of sodium chloride present?
    (A) 1 mOsm
    (B) 2 mOsm
    (C) 3 mOsm
    (D) None of the above

29. Osmotic activity is a function of
    (A) electrolytes only.
    (B) nonelectrolytes only.
    (C) strong electrolytes only.
    (D) the total number of particles present in solution.

30. If one assumes complete dissociation, how many milliosmols of sodium chloride are in 100 ml of a 0.9% solution?

    (A) 2 mOsm

    (B) 3 mOsm

    (C) 31 mOsm

    (D) 45 mOsm

31. Which of the following statements is false?

    (A) Hydrogen has one proton.

    (B) Hydrogen has one electron in the K shell.

    (C) Hydrogen has one neutron in its nucleus.

    (D) Hydrogen has an atomic number and an atomic weight of 1.

32. Beryllium has five neutrons and two electrons each in the K and L shell, respectively. Therefore, beryllium has an atomic weight of

    (A) 5 and an atomic number of 4.

    (B) 9 and an atomic number of 5.

    (C) 4 and an atomic number of 9.

    (D) 9 and an atomic number of 4.

33. The chemical symbol for mercury is Hg, whereas that for oxygen is O. If HgO is mercuric oxide, what is mercurous oxide?

    (A) HgO_2

    (B) Hg_2O

    (C) Hg_2O_3

    (D) Hg_3O_2

34. HNO_3 is the chemical formula for nitric acid; HNO_2 is the chemical formula for

    (A) nitrous acid.

    (B) nitronous acid.

    (C) nitrate acid.

    (D) nitrite acid.

35. The combination of an element A with an element B to form a new compound AB is called a synthetic reaction. The reverse of this reaction is called

    (A) single replacement.

    (B) synthesis.

    (C) decomposition.

    (D) double replacement.

36. Pick out the incorrect statement.

    (A) Oxidation is associated with the loss of electrons.

    (B) Oxidation-reduction reactions involve the loss and gain of electrons.

    (C) The oxidized particle (atom) shows a decrease in valence number.

    (D) Reduction involves the gain of electrons.

37. You are given the equation $ABC_3 \rightarrow AB + C_2$. The balanced equation is

    (A) $2ABC_3 \rightarrow AB + 3C_2$

    (B) $ABC_3 \rightarrow AB + C_2$

    (C) $2ABC_3 \rightarrow 2AB + 3C_2$

    (D) $3ABC_3 \rightarrow 3AB + 3C_2$

38. A molecule of oxygen contains two atoms of oxygen. How many atoms of oxygen does a molecule of ozone contain?

    (A) 2

    (B) 4

    (C) 1

    (D) 3

39. Which statement is false?

    (A) Oxygen burns by itself.

    (B) Oxygen is an odorless and colorless gas.

    (C) Oxygen supports combustion.

    (D) Air contains about 20% oxygen.

40. Hydrogen peroxide decomposes to yield

    (A) two molecules of water and two molecules of oxygen.

    (B) one molecule of water and one molecule of oxygen.

    (C) three molecules of water and two molecules of oxygen.

    (D) two molecules of water and one molecule of oxygen.

41. A volumetric flask contains 5,000 ml of water. What is the weight of this quantity of water?

    (A) 50 g

    (B) 500 g

    (C) 5,000 g

    (D) 50,000 g

42. Molarity (*M*) is best defined as moles of solute per

    (A) kiloliter of solution.

    (B) kilogram of solution.

    (C) 100 ml of solution.

    (D) liter of solution.

43. A total of 40 g of sodium hydroxide is dissolved in water to give a final volume of 400 ml. What is the molarity of this solution? (Na = 23, O = 16, H = 1)

    (A) 0.25 *M*

    (B) 2.5 *M*

    (C) 25 *M*

    (D) 0.1 *M*

44. How many moles of solute are there in 125 ml of a 5 *M* solution of sodium hydroxide?

    (A) 10.0 mol

    (B) 3.40 mol

    (C) 0.625 mol

    (D) 6.25 mol

45. How much sodium hydroxide is there in 125 ml of a 5 *M* solution of sodium hydroxide?

    (A) 75.0 g

    (B) 62.5 g

    (C) 25.0 g

    (D) 80.5 g

46. What is the molarity of 1 liter of pure water (H_2O)?

    (A) 55.5 *M*

    (B) 18 *M*

    (C) 19 *M*

    (D) It cannot be determined.

47. All of the following are colligative properties of solutions EXCEPT the

    (A) boiling point.

    (B) vapor pressure.

    (C) freezing point.

    (D) specific gravity.

48. Given that the hydrogen ion concentration (moles per liter) of a solution is 1.0, what is its pH?

    (A) 0

    (B) 1

    (C) 7

    (D) 14

49. Given the same hydrogen ion concentration (in moles/liter) of 1.0, calculate the pH value of this solution.

    (A) 0

    (B) 1

    (C) 7

    (D) 14

50. The higher the pH of a solution, the

    (A) lower the acidity.

    (B) higher the hydrogen ion concentration.

    (C) lower the basicity.

    (D) stronger the acid.

51. Which of the following statements is false?

    (A) Methane is important in addition reactions.

    (B) Methane is explosive when combined with air.

    (C) Methane is a major component of natural gas.

    (D) Methane is commonly known as marsh gas.

52. All of the following are esters EXCEPT

    (A) ethyl acetate.

    (B) methyl salicylate.

    (C) sodium formate.

    (D) nitroglycerine.

53. Carbohydrates are compounds containing carbon, hydrogen, and oxygen. Which of the following is NOT a carbohydrate?

    (A) Glucose

    (B) Glyceryl stearate

    (C) Dextran

    (D) Cellulose

54. Pick out the nonsynthetic fiber.

    (A) Cellulose

    (B) Rayon

    (C) Orlon

    (D) Nylon

55. The uncertainty principle, which states that it is impossible to know with exactitude both the momentum and position of an electron simultaneously, is associated with

    (A) Heisenberg.

    (B) Planck.

    (C) de Broglie.

    (D) Bohr.

56. How many quantum numbers are necessary in order to define electronic wave functions?

    (A) 4

    (B) 3

    (C) 2

    (D) 1

57. Wolfgang Pauli's exclusion principle states that

    (A) no two electrons in an atom can have the same three quantum numbers.

    (B) no two electrons in an atom can have the same four quantum numbers.

    (C) no two electrons can have the same orbital.

    (D) any two electrons in an atom can have the same four quantum numbers.

58. The electronic distribution in the orbitals of an oxygen atom is

    (A) $1s^2 2s^4 2p^2$

    (B) $1s^2 2s^2 2p^4$

    (C) $1s^2 2s^2 2p^8$

    (D) $1s^2 2s^2 2p^6$

59. Carbon has 6 protons, and its atomic weight is 12. How many electrons and neutrons does it have?

    (A) 3 electrons, 9 neutrons

    (B) 6 electrons, 6 neutrons

    (C) 6 electrons, 12 neutrons

    (D) It cannot be determined.

60. Name the element with the electronic distribution $1s^2 2s^2 2p^2$:

    (A) Helium

    (B) Carbon

    (C) Beryllium

    (D) Oxygen

61. Isotopes are atoms of elements differing only in

    (A) valence.

    (B) the number of electrons.

    (C) chemical property.

    (D) mass.

62. Carbon-14 is a commonly used radioisotope in medical research. How many more neutrons does it have compared to natural carbon?

    (A) 2

    (B) 4

    (C) 6

    (D) 0

63. Pick out the statement about gamma-ray decay that is false.

    (A) The number of protons does not change.

    (B) It results in a decrease of 4 units of atomic mass.

    (C) There is emission of photons.

    (D) The number of neutrons does not change.

64. Electromagnetic radiation has a wide spectrum of energies and wavelengths. The angstrom is widely used as a unit to measure wavelength. What does it equal in meters?

    (A) 1×10^{-15} m

    (B) 1×10^{-9} m

    (C) 1×10^{-10} m

    (D) 1×10^{-11} m

65. Pyrophosphoric acid is $H_4P_2O_7$. What does the prefix *pyro-* indicate?

    (A) Lowest oxidation state

    (B) Highest oxidation state

    (C) Highest hydrated form

    (D) Loss of water

66. Lead (Pb) has many industrial uses. Lead ion exists in two oxidation states, which are

    (A) divalent and tetravalent.

    (B) monovalent and trivalent.

    (C) divalent and pentavalent.

    (D) monovalent and divalent.

67. Plaster of paris is made by heating gypsum until it loses three fourths of its water of hydration. What alkaline-earth metal is found in gypsum and plaster of paris?

    (A) Phosphorus

    (B) Calcium

    (C) Magnesium

    (D) Barium

68. Hydrogen sulfide (H_2S) can be prepared by the action of an acid on any metallic sulfide. All of the following are characteristics of hydrogen sulfide EXCEPT

    (A) colorless gas.

    (B) denser than air.

    (C) nontoxic.

    (D) odor of rotten eggs.

69. What is the common name for the organic acid with the formula CH_3COOH?

    (A) Aqua fortis

    (B) Muriatic acid

    (C) Aqua regia

    (D) Vinegar

70. If table salt is sodium chloride, which of the following is the formula for baking soda?

    (A) $Na_2B_4O_7$

    (B) $MgSO_4$

    (C) Na_2CO_3

    (D) $NaHCO_3$

71. HOCl is a more powerful oxidizing agent than chlorine. What is HOCl?

    (A) Tincture of iodine

    (B) Chloroform

    (C) Hypochlorous acid

    (D) Brine

72. Alkenes do NOT possess a(n)

    (A) pi bond.

    (B) alpha bond.

    (C) double bond.

    (D) sigma bond.

73. Amino acids are generally represented by the formula RNH_2COOH. What class of organic compounds is represented by $RCONH_2$?

    (A) Amides

    (B) Esters

    (C) Amines

    (D) Azides

74. In chemistry, the suffix *-ase*, as in lipase, denotes a(n)

    (A) carboxyl group.

    (B) base.

    (C) enzyme.

    (D) sugar.

75. A primary alcohol has at least two hydrogens attached to the alcohol carbon. A tertiary alcohol has

    (A) no hydrogens attached to the alcohol carbon.

    (B) only hydrogen attached to the alcohol carbon.

    (C) three hydrogens attached to the alcohol carbon.

    (D) only one hydrogen attached to the alcohol carbon.

76. Which of the formulas below is methyl vinyl ketone?

    (A) $CH_3OCH_2CH = CH_2$

    (B) $CH_3COCH = CH_2$

    (C) $CH_3CH_2CH_2 = COOH$

    (D) $CH_3CH_2COCH = CH_2$

77. The incorrect way of naming an organic acid is by

    (A) using the hydrocarbon name of the longest chain.

    (B) designating the carboxyl carbon as carbon number 1.

    (C) changing the suffix from *-ane* to *anoic*.

    (D) changing the suffix from *-ane* to *-ol*.

78. Name the hydrocarbon, $CH_3(CH_2)_8CH_3$.

    (A) Nonane

    (B) Octane

    (C) Undecane

    (D) Decane

79. Pick out the incorrect statement.

    (A) Atoms connected by single bonds rotate around the bond.

    (B) Atoms in double bonds are not free to rotate.

    (C) Atoms in a ring are free to rotate around their bonds.

    (D) Atoms in triple bonds are not free to rotate.

80. Pick out the incorrect statement.

    (A) The stability of a carbonium ion is increased by charge dispersal.

    (B) A primary carbonium ion forms more easily than a tertiary carbonium ion.

    (C) The carbon atom in a carbonium ion has only 6 electrons.

    (D) Carbonium ions can be classified as primary, secondary, or tertiary.

81. With regard to benzene, which one of the following statements is incorrect?

    (A) It is a flat (planar) molecule.

    (B) It has the formula C_6H_6.

    (C) It is a symmetrical molecule.

    (D) It has a bond angle of 150°.

82. With regard to the carbonyl carbons of aldehydes and ketones, which one of the following statements is false?

    (A) They usually have a bond angle of 120°.

    (B) They are oriented such that carbon and oxygen are joined by a double bond.

    (C) They are sp^2 hybridized and not planar.

    (D) They are connected to three other atoms by sigma bonds.

83. Nucleophilic substitution is commonly encountered in organic chemistry. Select the one statement below that is correct, concerning nucleophilic displacement.

    (A) Amines are more reactive than amides.

    (B) Acid chlorides are more reactive than alkyl chloride.

    (C) Ethers are more reactive than esters.

    (D) Saturated carbons are more reactive than acyl carbon.

84. Glycols are

    (A) alcohols containing two hydroxyl groups.

    (B) alcohols without any hydroxyl group.

    (C) aldehydes containing two hydroxyl groups.

    (D) ketones containing two hydroxyl groups.

85. The Grignard reagent is very useful in organic chemistry. Pick out the one incorrect statement about it.

    (A) Its general name is alkylmagnesium halide.

    (B) The magnesium-halogen bond is covalent.

    (C) The carbon-magnesium bond is considered covalent.

    (D) Its general formula is RMgX.

86. Which is the correct statement?

    (A) Optically inactive reactants yield optically active products.

    (B) Optically active products are the result of optically inactive reactants.

    (C) Optically inactive reactants yield optically inactive products.

    (D) The preparation of dissymmetric compounds from symmetric reactants yields no racemic modification.

87. If CH_4 is methane, what is CH_2?

    (A) Methanol

    (B) Mesyl

    (C) Methyl

    (D) Methylene

88. The Diels-Alder reaction does NOT involve

    (A) a diene and a dienophile.

    (B) a product that is six-membered.

    (C) αβ-unsaturated carbonyl compounds.

    (D) electron-releasing groups in the dienophile.

89. Disaccharides are composed of two monosaccharide units. Which of the following is NOT a disaccharide?

    (A) Amylose

    (B) Lactose

    (C) Maltose

    (D) Sucrose

90. Which of the following amino acids is simplest in structure?

   (A) Arginine

   (B) Tyrosine

   (C) Glycine

   (D) Methionine

91. Aryl halides are compounds containing halogen attached

   (A) to a side chain of an aromatic ring.

   (B) directly to an aromatic ring.

   (C) directly to a cyclic alkane.

   (D) to an alkene.

92. Ethylene oxide is best described as an

   (A) alkane.

   (B) alkene.

   (C) aldehyde.

   (D) epoxide.

93. Amines may have all of the following formulas EXCEPT

   (A) RNH_2

   (B) R_3N

   (C) RNH

   (D) R_2NH

94. Absolute alcohol is

   (A) a mixture of fifty parts of alcohol to water.

   (B) 80% alcohol.

   (C) water-free alcohol.

   (D) wood alcohol.

95. Two aromatic rings sharing a pair of carbon atoms are called fused-ring hydrocarbons. The simplest member of this family of compounds is

   (A) naphthalene.

   (B) phenanthrene.

   (C) benzene.

   (D) anthracene.

96. CH_3OH is usually known as

   (A) menthone.

   (B) methanol.

   (C) menthol.

   (D) mesitol.

97. All the following describes Tollen's reagent EXCEPT

   (A) reduction of silver ion to free silver.

   (B) oxidation of an aldehyde.

   (C) reduction of an acid to aldehyde.

   (D) silver ammonia ion.

98. In forming ammonia, nitrogen uses

   (A) sp orbitals.

   (B) sp^1 orbitals.

   (C) sp^2 orbitals.

   (D) sp^3 orbitals.

99. An acid chloride can be prepared by substitution of the hydroxyl group of a carboxylic acid. The following reagents are commonly used to prepare acid chlorides EXCEPT

   (A) thionyl chloride.

   (B) ethyl chloride.

   (C) phosphorus trichloride.

   (D) phosphorus pentachloride.

100. Which is the incorrect statement?

   (A) Sucrose is a reducing sugar.

   (B) All monosaccharides are reducing sugars.

   (C) Glucose is a monosaccharide.

   (D) Glucose is a reducing sugar.

VERBAL ABILITY

70 Questions • 60 Minutes

Directions: Choose the word that best completes the analogy.

1. CARDINAL : PRIMARY ::
   SECONDARY :
   (A) tertiary
   (B) subordinate
   (C) pivotal
   (D) key

2. AWAKE : ALIVE :: ASLEEP :
   (A) arouse
   (B) defunct
   (C) functional
   (D) excited

3. TACT : SAVOIR FAIRE :: COARSE :
   (A) act
   (B) diplomacy
   (C) crude
   (D) expert

4. EXPERT : ADEPT :: AMATEUR :
   (A) dabbler
   (B) beginner
   (C) authority
   (D) crackerjack

5. ACCOUNT : DEEM ::
   UNDERVALUE :
   (A) consider
   (B) regard
   (C) view
   (D) depreciate

6. SEQUELA : RESULT :: PRIMARY :
   (A) secondary
   (B) end
   (C) after effect
   (D) basis

7. BULLETIN : BOARD ::
   ANNOUNCEMENT :
   (A) mail
   (B) telephone
   (C) newt
   (D) bullet

8. BRIDLE : RESTRAIN :: JAIL :
   (A) bridge
   (B) marry
   (C) lockup
   (D) center

9. CONTAMINATE : POLLUTE ::
   WRECK :
   (A) crash
   (B) contemplate
   (C) contain
   (D) purify

10. DISPLEASURE : PIQUE ::
    PLEASURE :
    (A) joy
    (B) disposal
    (C) madness
    (D) bitterness

11. EVENTUATE : ENSUE ::
    UNDOUBTED :
    (A) end
    (B) entwine
    (C) crease
    (D) authentic

12. MAGNIFICENCE : GRANDIOSITY ::
    SCHNOOK :
    (A) fame
    (B) magnifier
    (C) dunce
    (D) magnitude

13. UNDULATE : STILL :: RETREAT :
    (A) poll
    (B) charge
    (C) free
    (D) retch

14. PARSIMONIOUS : SCROOGE ::
    LINCOLN :
    (A) miserly
    (B) liberal
    (C) conservative
    (D) genuine

15. QUIESCENT : DORMANT ::
    MOBILE :
    (A) auto
    (B) running
    (C) plane
    (D) quick

16. RADIOACTIVITY : RADIATION ::
    RADIO :
    (A) frequency
    (B) place
    (C) radar
    (D) ion

17. DEAN : STUDENT :: WIFE :
    (A) group
    (B) associate
    (C) son
    (D) relative

18. FLANK : END :: FEET :
    (A) side
    (B) meter
    (C) head
    (D) inches

19. DIPSOMANIAC : ALCOHOL ::
    ADDICT :
    (A) diplomat
    (B) insomniac
    (C) addiction
    (D) morphine

20. CORSAGE : NOSEGAY :: BUTLER :
    (A) maid
    (B) valet
    (C) receptionist
    (D) corset

21. CORTEGE : RETINUE :: LANE :
    (A) roadway
    (B) median
    (C) line
    (D) lineation

22. JOWL : JAW :: PIG :
    (A) head
    (B) cow
    (C) porcine
    (D) mule

23. SURMOUNT : CONQUER :: VICTORY :
    (A) survey
    (B) conquest
    (C) suspect
    (D) recount

24. PLIABLE : FLEXIBLE :: AGILE :
    (A) supple
    (B) scrupulous
    (C) programmable
    (D) reliable

25. ZEAL : INDIFFERENCE :: FERVOR :
    (A) foolishness
    (B) bright
    (C) pleasure
    (D) mute

26. TRANSCEND : LAG :: DUNCE :
    (A) overtake
    (B) pass
    (C) exceed
    (D) brainy

27. SHREWD : CALCULATING :: ODD :
    (A) cagey
    (B) strange
    (C) shrinkable
    (D) even

28. EXPENDITURE : DISBURSEMENT ::
    OVOLO :
    (A) credit
    (B) molding
    (C) debit
    (D) roe

29. EXPEDIENCY : RESOURCE ::
    EXPECT :
    (A) excellence
    (B) expulsion
    (C) efficiency
    (D) count

30. BEGUILE : DECEIVE :: DEPART :
    (A) become
    (B) envy
    (C) withdraw
    (D) enrage

31. EXODUS : BOOK :: BATMAN :
    (A) comics
    (B) radio
    (C) television
    (D) report

32. DENOUNCE : EULOGIZE ::
    PRODIGALITY :
    (A) parsimonious
    (B) impeach
    (C) connote
    (D) express

33. DENUDE : PEEL :: PROGRESS :
    (A) headway
    (B) cancel
    (C) depart
    (D) depress

34. CIRCUMSCRIBE : LIMIT ::
    PROGRAMMA :
    (A) chasten
    (B) circulate
    (C) agenda
    (D) launch

35. DEVIANT : NORMAL :: STARVE :
    (A) aberrant
    (B) suckle
    (C) nontitled
    (D) ghostly

36. MELEE : SKIRMISH :: INNING :
    (A) agreement
    (B) melange
    (C) frame
    (D) merger

37. ENIGMA : MYSTERY :: NOVEL :
    (A) enemy
    (B) neoteric
    (C) mark
    (D) imprecation

38. PALPABLE : TOUCHABLE :: SOFT :
    - **(A)** pulpy
    - **(B)** pristine
    - **(C)** hard
    - **(D)** tactful

39. RUDIMENTARY : ELEMENTAL :: RUDE :
    - **(A)** parcel
    - **(B)** civil
    - **(C)** urbane
    - **(D)** crude

40. IMPUGN : DESTROY :: LOVED :
    - **(A)** deny
    - **(B)** adored
    - **(C)** implant
    - **(D)** return

41. VALIDATE : ABROGATE : CONFIRM :
    - **(A)** contradict
    - **(B)** accede
    - **(C)** assent
    - **(D)** validate

42. TARIFF : DUTY :: TAUNT :
    - **(A)** post
    - **(B)** slack
    - **(C)** goal
    - **(D)** deride

43. WASTREL : VANGUARD :: MISER :
    - **(A)** vagrant
    - **(B)** spendthrift
    - **(C)** wrangler
    - **(D)** straggler

44. YAHOO : RUFFIAN :: MILKSOP :
    - **(A)** yak
    - **(B)** doormat
    - **(C)** macho
    - **(D)** gravy

45. SUAVE : URBANE :: RAMPART :
    - **(A)** blues
    - **(B)** foolish
    - **(C)** bastion
    - **(D)** urban

46. REMORSELESS : IMPENITENT :: IMPEND :
    - **(A)** loom
    - **(B)** remorseful
    - **(C)** impatient
    - **(D)** regretful

47. PERSNICKETY : FASTIDIOUS :: PERSUADABLE :
    - **(A)** easy
    - **(B)** pernicious
    - **(C)** chancy
    - **(D)** receptive

48. PERIMETER : INNERMORE :: EXTERNAL :
    - **(A)** period
    - **(B)** internal
    - **(C)** area
    - **(D)** end zone

49. IMPERIOUS : GENTLE :: GROVELING :
    - **(A)** kindly
    - **(B)** domineering
    - **(C)** considerate
    - **(D)** domestic

50. COMPASSION : SYMPATHY :: DOODLE :
    - **(A)** unconcern
    - **(B)** implacability
    - **(C)** relentlessness
    - **(D)** imbecile

FOR QUESTIONS 51–70, CHOOSE THE WORD OR SET OF WORDS THAT BEST COMPLETES THE SENTENCE.

51. It is _____ that students do not repay their student loans and thereby make it more _____ for future generations of students to obtain them.

    (A) unfortunate .. urgent

    (B) regrettable .. difficult

    (C) unforgivable .. likely

    (D) laudable .. practical

52. Although her initial success was _____ by the fact that she was the daughter of a famous actor, the critics later _____ her as a star in her own right.

    (A) enhanced .. acclaimed

    (B) impeded .. criticized

    (C) refuted .. summarily acknowledged

    (D) superseded .. disavowed

53. Contrary to popular belief, the Mayans were not peace-loving astronomers but _____ warriors who viewed their gods as cruel and _____.

    (A) formidable .. vengeful

    (B) skilled .. benevolent

    (C) reluctant .. omnipotent

    (D) docile .. patronizing

54. Despite the fact that she was much _____, the scientist continued to present her controversial theories to the _____ of the Royal Academy, whose members repeatedly denounced her research.

    (A) admired .. chagrin

    (B) revered .. benefit

    (C) imitated .. foreboding

    (D) maligned .. consternation

55. Washington Irving, the father of American literature and creator of such delightful characters as Ichabod Crane and Rip Van Winkle, will be remembered more for the _____ of his prose than for the originality of his tales, which were _____ from popular folklore.

    (A) density .. obtained

    (B) vulgarity .. stolen

    (C) mediocrity .. descended

    (D) charm .. borrowed

56. Although alcoholism has long been regarded as a personality disorder, there is evidence to suggest that alcoholics are often children of alcoholics and that they are born with a _____ the disease.

    (A) respect for

    (B) predisposition to

    (C) liability for

    (D) deterioration of

57. Despite the millions of dollars spent on improvements, the telephone system in India remains _____ and continues to _____ the citizens who depend on it.

    (A) primitive .. inconvenience

    (B) bombastic .. upset

    (C) suspicious .. connect

    (D) outdated .. elate

58. Contrary to popular opinion, bats are not generally aggressive and rabid; most are shy and _____.

    (A) turgid

    (B) disfigured

    (C) punctual

    (D) innocuous

59. Unlike the images in symbolist poetry which are often vague and _____, the images of surrealist poetry are startlingly _____ and bold.

    (A) extraneous .. furtive

    (B) trivial .. inadvertent

    (C) obscure .. concrete

    (D) spectacular .. pallid

60. A good trial lawyer will argue only what is central to an issue, eliminating _____ information or anything else that might _____ the client.

    (A) seminal .. amuse

    (B) extraneous .. jeopardize

    (C) erratic .. enhance

    (D) prodigious .. extol

61. Psychologists and science fiction writers argue that people persist in believing in extraterrestrial life, even though the federal government _____ all such beliefs, because people need to feel a personal sense of _____ in a godless universe.

    (A) decries .. morbidity

    (B) endorses .. despair

    (C) creates .. guilt

    (D) discourages .. spirituality

62. Pollen grains and spores that are 200 million years old are now being extracted from shale and are _____ the theory that the breakup of the continents occurred in stages; in fact, it seems that the breakups occurred almost _____.

    (A) refining .. blatantly

    (B) reshaping ... simultaneously

    (C) countermanding .. imperceptibly

    (D) forging .. vicariously

63. Because he was _____ and the life of the party, his friends thought that he was happy; but his wife was _____ and shy and was thought to be unhappy.

    (A) melancholy .. sympathetic

    (B) philanthropic .. conciliatory

    (C) vitriolic .. sophomoric

    (D) garrulous .. taciturn

64. His offhand, rather _____ remarks _____ a character that was really rather serious and not at all superficial.

    (A) flippant .. masked

    (B) pernicious .. betrayed

    (C) bellicose .. belied

    (D) controversial .. revealed

65. Although the faculty did not always agree with the chairperson of the department, they _____ her ideas, mostly in _____ her seniority and out of respect for her previous achievements.

    (A) scoffed at .. fear of

    (B) harbored .. defense of

    (C) implemented .. deference to

    (D) marveled at .. lieu of

66. Psychologists agree that human beings have a strong need to _____ their time; having too much idle time can be as stressful as having none at all.

    (A) threaten

    (B) annihilate

    (C) structure

    (D) punctuate

67. While scientists continue to make advances in the field of _____, some members of the clergy continue to oppose the research, arguing that it is _____ for human beings to tamper with life.

    (A) psychology .. imperative
    (B) astronomy .. fallacious
    (C) genetics .. immoral
    (D) geology .. erroneous

68. Although for centuries literature was considered something that would instruct as well as entertain, the modern reader has little patience with _____ works and seeks only to be _____.

    (A) epic .. demoralized
    (B) didactic .. distracted
    (C) bawdy .. absorbed
    (D) superficial .. enlightened

69. Because of the _____ of acupuncture therapy in China, Western physicians are starting to learn the procedure.

    (A) veracity
    (B) manipulation
    (C) liquidity
    (D) effectiveness

70. The conclusion of the program was a modern symphony with chords so _____ that the piece produced sound similar to the _____ one hears as the individual orchestra members tune their instruments before a concert.

    (A) superfluous .. melody
    (B) discordant .. cacophony
    (C) melodious .. applause
    (D) versatile .. harmony

CRITICAL THINKING ESSAY

Time—30 Minutes

Directions: In this section, you will have 30 minutes to analyze and explain your views on one of the topics presented below. Read the statement carefully. Write only on one of the topics given.

Argumentative Topic:

How have changes to the U.S. health-care system affected you or members of your family?

Problem-Solving Topic:

What process improvements would you suggest be made to the Medicare Prescription Drug Plan?

ANSWER KEY AND EXPLANATIONS

Reading Comprehension

1.	D	11.	C	21.	D	31.	B	41.	B
2.	B	12.	C	22.	B	32.	A	42.	B
3.	A	13.	A	23.	B	33.	D	43.	B
4.	B	14.	D	24.	C	34.	C	44.	C
5.	D	15.	B	25.	C	35.	C	45.	B
6.	B	16.	A	26.	B	36.	B	46.	C
7.	C	17.	C	27.	A	37.	A	47.	B
8.	B	18.	C	28.	C	38.	D	48.	D
9.	C	19.	B	29.	B	39.	C		
10.	D	20.	B	30.	D	40.	A		

1. **The correct answer is (D).** The answer to this question is found in lines 7 and 8 of the paragraph. An intramuscular solution is given intramuscularly rather than intravenously.

2. **The correct answer is (B).** The answer is found in lines 20–24 of the paragraph. There are several variables, including the answer, that affect the rate of flow of medication: gravity, temperature, and possibly the equipment itself.

3. **The correct answer is (A).** The answer is found in lines 26–30: "When the rate of flow is critical, such as in pediatric patients or in parenteral nutrition, an infusion pump may be needed to ensure the proper flow of solution into the patient."

4. **The correct answer is (B).** The answer is found in lines 1–4 of the paragraph: "Before the intravenous administration of a medication, it is essential to check the medication, the dose, fluid in which the drug is to be given, and time of administration against the patient's chart."

5. **The correct answer is (D).** The answer is found in lines 24–26 of the paragraph: "…it should be checked every hour or so, depending on hospital policy."

6. **The correct answer is (B).** The answer is found in lines 1–3 of the paragraph. Bronchoconstrictors do not appear in the list of items in which adrenergic agents are commonly found.

7. **The correct answer is (C).** The answer is found in lines 19–21 of the paragraph: "General anesthetics producing parasympathetic and sympathetic imbalance may cause pupillary block."

8. **The correct answer is (B).** The answer is found in lines 13–18 of the paragraph: "It is important to note, however, that these agents will elevate the intraocular pressure by narrowing the anterior chamber angle when instilled into eyes of angle closure patients."

9. **The correct answer is (C).** The answer is found in lines 10–13 of the paragraph: "Adrenergic agents such as epinephrine and phenylephrine have been used ocularly to treat open-angle glaucoma."

10. **The correct answer is (D).** The answer is found in lines 21–24 of the paragraph: "To prevent this complication, topical pilocarpine at 1% may be instilled into the eye 1 hour prior to anesthesia."

11. **The correct answer is (C).** The answer is found in lines 7–9 of the paragraph: "Ventricular tachycardia usually requires intravenous therapy."

12. **The correct answer is (C).** The answer is found in lines 17–20 of the paragraph: "Doses of 50–100 mg of diphenylhydantoin, up to a maximum of 1.0 g, may be administered intravenously every 5 minutes. . . ."

13. **The correct answer is (A).** The answer is found in lines 27–29 of the paragraph: "Generally, cardiovascular complications can be avoided with an infusion rate of 20–50 mg/min."

14. **The correct answer is (D).** The answer is found in lines 22–26 of the paragraph: "Single intravenous doses of 300 mg or more produce a more marked hypotension (20–45 mmHg) and also lead to subtherapeutic diphenylhydantoin plasma levels. . . ."

15. **The correct answer is (B).** The answer is found in lines 9–13 of the paragraph: "There appears to be no indication in this situation for intramuscular injections, because the drug is slowly and erratically absorbed from the site, besides being very painful."

16. **The correct answer is (A).** The answer is found in lines 1–3 of the paragraph: "In open-angle glaucoma, a physical blockage occurs within the trabecular meshwork that retards elimination. . . ."

17. **The correct answer is (C).** The answer is found in line 10 of the paragraph. The normal intraocular pressure is 10–20 mmHg.

18. **The correct answer is (C).** The answer is found in lines 14 and 15 of the paragraph. Visual field effects occur eventually and only after the disease has been present for a period of time. The changes are not immediate.

19. **The correct answer is (B).** The answer is found in lines 8–10 of the paragraph: "The impairment of aqueous drainage elevates the intraocular pressure (IOP) to 25–35 mmHg. . . ."

20. **The correct answer is (B).** The answer is found in lines 4–6 of the paragraph: "The obstruction is presumed to be located between the trabecular sheet and the episcleral veins. . . ."

21. **The correct answer is (D).** The answer is found in lines 2–4 of the paragraph: "Besides loss of consciousness, these syncopal attacks involve pallor, muscular twitching, and sometimes seizures."

22. **The correct answer is (B).** The answer is found in lines 22–26 of the paragraph: "An adverse dose-related effect is hypotension, which may occur by alpha-adrenergic receptor blockade or by a direct negative inotropic effect on the heart."

23. **The correct answer is (B).** The answer is found in lines 5–7 of the paragraph: "When an EKG is obtained during an attack, the pattern indicates ventricular tachyarrhythmia. . . ."

24. **The correct answer is (C).** The answer is found in line 1 of the paragraph: "An unusual reaction to quinidine is syncope."

25. **The correct answer is (C).** The answer is found in lines 19–21 of the paragraph: "Syncope may occur at low doses (e.g., 0.8 g/day). . . ."

26. **The correct answer is (B).** The answer is found in lines 1–4 of the paragraph: "Many reports have indicated that the tricyclic antidepressants, especially imipramine, may be of benefit in the treatment of MBD in children."

27. **The correct answer is (A).** The answer is found in lines 12–14 of the paragraph: ". . . the maximum daily dose approved by the FDA (5 mg/kg per day) . . ."

28. **The correct answer is (C).** The answer is found in lines 4–7 of the paragraph: "However, although most studies have indicated their superiority over placebos, they are still not as effective as the psychostimulants."

29. **The correct answer is (B).** The answer is found in lines 18–21 of the paragraph: "In addition, the patient should be monitored for more severe effects on the central nervous system, for example, seizures. . . ."

30. **The correct answer is (D).** The answer is found in lines 8–11 of the paragraph: "Further drawbacks associated with their use include the development of tolerance in some children and numerous deleterious side effects."

31. **The correct answer is (B).** The answer is found in lines 10–12 of the paragraph: "Dextroamphetamine was initially used in 1937 and continued to be the agent of choice until the late 1960s. . . ."

32. **The correct answer is (A).** The answer is found in lines 23–26 of the paragraph: " . . . while proponents of dextroamphetamine indicate that, in their hands, it has comparable clinical efficacy at a lower cost."

33. **The correct answer is (D).** The answer is found in lines 1–5 of the paragraph: "The primary agents in the treatment of MBD are the centrally acting sympathomimetics, for example, methylphenidate, dextroamphetamine, and magnesium pemoline."

34. **The correct answer is (C).** The answer is found in lines 12–15 of the paragraph: ". . .methylphenidate usage increased in association with reports of a lower incidence of side effects with the latter drug."

35. **The correct answer is (C).** The answer is found in lines 15–18 of the paragraph: "It would appear that these reports of the greater safety of methylphenidate therapy are of questionable clinical significance."

36. **The correct answer is (B).** The answer is found in lines 1 and 2 of the paragraph: "Procainamide may be considered as an alternative to quinidine. . . ."

37. **The correct answer is (A).** The answer is found in lines 15–18 of the paragraph: "Giardina et al. have intravenously administered 100 mg., up to a maximum of 1 g, every 5 minutes to treat ventricular arrhythmia."

38. **The correct answer is (D).** The answer is found in lines 13 and 14 of the paragraph: "Procainamide may be given intravenously at a rate of 25–50 mg/min."

39. **The correct answer is (C).** The answer is found in lines 4 and 5 of the paragraph: "Most patients absorb 75–95% of an oral dose. . . ."

40. **The correct answer is (A).** The answer is found in lines 5–7 of the paragraph: ". . .however, Koch-Weser estimated that 10% of subjects may absorb 50% or less."

41. **The correct answer is (B).** The answer is found in lines 16–19 of the paragraph: "The increase in intraocular pressure is approximately 10 mmHg for patients with preglaucomatous anterior chambers. . . ."

42. **The correct answer is (B).** The answer is found in lines 13–16 of the paragraph: "This ocular hypertensive effect is usually fully reversible within one month after discontinuation of steroid therapy."

43. **The correct answer is (B).** The answer is found in lines 20–23 of the paragraph: "In some cases, irreversible eye damage occurs if ocular tension persists for one to two months or longer."

44. The correct answer is (C). The answer is found in lines 2–4 of the paragraph: "This form of glaucoma is usually painless and involves no ocular findings or visual field defects."

45. The correct answer is (B). The answer is found in lines 27–30 of the paragraph: "Patients undergoing chronic topical steroid therapy should therefore have a tonometric examination every two months."

46. The correct answer is (C). This is a logical structure question that asks about the overall development of the selection. The main organizational principle of the passage is the comparison and contrast of art and knowledge. The author points to both similarities and differences between the two. Choice (A) is incorrect. Though the author proposes a theory of the purpose of art, there is no refutation of anything in the passage. As for choice (B), the author offers some general conclusions, but makes no generalizations based on examples. As for choice (D), though the passage can be viewed as an answer to the question "What is art for?" the author does not make question and answer the organizational principle of the selection.

47. The correct answer is (B). This is a specific detail question, so the correct answer will be explicitly stated in the selection. Choice (B) is specifically stated. The author states that the knowledge of prior generations is preserved in speech. So knowledge is cumulative. Later, the author states that knowledge is self-correcting; that is, that errors are, during the passing of time, eliminated. So knowledge is also progressive.

48. The correct answer is (D). This is a specific detail question. The author specifically says that art is communication (like words), so choice (A) is mentioned. The author also states that art has the function of producing loftier emotions, so choice (B) is mentioned. And the author says that art renders the experience of previous generations accessible to the present, so choice (C) is mentioned. Choice (D), however, is not said by the author to be true of art. In fact, in the last sentence, the author strongly implies that art can be bad as well as good.

Biology

1.	C	16.	A	31.	A	46.	B	61.	C
2.	B	17.	B	32.	D	47.	A	62.	A
3.	B	18.	C	33.	B	48.	C	63.	D
4.	C	19.	D	34.	B	49.	D	64.	B
5.	D	20.	B	35.	C	50.	A	65.	C
6.	D	21.	D	36.	D	51.	D	66.	D
7.	B	22.	A	37.	C	52.	C	67.	C
8.	A	23.	D	38.	A	53.	C	68.	A
9.	A	24.	C	39.	D	54.	A	69.	B
10.	C	25.	B	40.	D	55.	A	70.	D
11.	D	26.	C	41.	A	56.	D	71.	C
12.	B	27.	C	42.	C	57.	B	72.	D
13.	A	28.	D	43.	C	58.	C	73.	A
14.	C	29.	A	44.	B	59.	D	74.	C
15.	B	30.	C	45.	C	60.	A	75.	A

1. **The correct answer is (C).** The cell is the smallest unit of life that can survive independently. The gene of a cell resides in the nucleus of the cell and can be considered an organelle or part of the cellular machinery. An organ is composed of living cells.

2. **The correct answer is (B).** The mitochondria is the primary source of energy for the aerobic cell. The endoplasmic reticulum and Golgi apparatus use energy from the mitochondria to synthesize and store cellular products. The nucleus is primarily responsible for the storage of genetic information.

3. **The correct answer is (B).** By using a Punnett square, we see that two *Bb* individuals have a 1-in-4 (25%) chance of producing an offspring with blue (*bb*) eyes.

	B	*b*
B	*BB*	*Bb*
b	*Bb*	*bb*

4. **The correct answer is (C).** Hypertonic solutions have a greater salt, or electrolyte, concentration than do red blood cells. Therefore, water leaves blood cells and enters the hypertonic solution, causing the red blood cells to shrink. Both isotonic and iso-osmotic solutions will have no effect on the red blood cells. A hypotonic solution will cause water to enter the red blood cells because of their higher electrolyte concentration and cause the cells to swell.

5. **The correct answer is (D).** Copper is considered a trace element that is necessary for normal metabolism of the body. Sodium, potassium, and calcium are major elements vital to the healthy body.

6. **The correct answer is (D).** A cross between a homozygous brown individual (*BB*) and a homozygous white individual (*bb*) will result in all offspring being brown heterozygous (*Bb*), as seen in the Punnett square.

	B	*B*
b	*Bb*	*Bb*
b	*Bb*	*Bb*

7. **The correct answer is (B).** Vitamins A, D, E, and K are fat-soluble vitamins. All the B vitamins, as well as vitamin C, are water-soluble vitamins.

8. **The correct answer is (A).** Under basal conditions, the liver receives about 25 percent of the total cardiac output, whereas the brain and skeletal muscle receive about 15 percent. The bone is relatively nonvascularized and receives only 5 percent of the total blood flow.

9. **The correct answer is (A).** Sodium is the most abundant electrolyte in extracellular fluid (~142 mEq/liter) with potassium the most abundant electrolyte (~141 mEq/liter) inside the cell (intracellular fluid). Both calcium (0–5 mEq/liter) and magnesium (3–58 mEq/liter) exist in relatively small amounts in the extracellular fluid.

10. **The correct answer is (C).** The small intestine has the largest surface area and carries out most of the specialized transport mechanisms in the gastrointestinal tract. Very little absorption of nutrients occurs in the stomach or the large intestine, also referred to as the colon.

11. **The correct answer is (D).** Long-chain (more than 10 carbons) fatty acids normally enter the circulatory system by way of the lymphatic system, packaged as chylomicrons. Short-chain fatty acids normally enter the circulatory system directly as free fatty acids.

12. **The correct answer is (B).** See the explanation for Answer 9.

13. **The correct answer is (A).** Scurvy is a disease resulting from a vitamin C deficiency. Deficiencies in thiamine, niacin, and vitamin D result in beriberi, pellagra, and rickets, respectively.

14. **The correct answer is (C).** Squamous epithelium is normally associated with body surfaces, as a form of protection (i.e., skin). Epithelium associated with the kidney, lungs, and pancreas is more suited for secretory functions and is columnar or cuboidal in nature.

15. **The correct answer is (B).** Chromatin is composed of DNA and protein and is found primarily in the nucleus.

16. **The correct answer is (A).** Skeletal muscle fibers contract and relax in about 0.1 second. Cardiac muscle requires 1–5 seconds, whereas smooth muscle needs more than 3 seconds to contract and relax.

17. **The correct answer is (B).** Saturated fats have all their carbon bonds saturated with hydrogens; thus, there are no double bonds. As the number of double bonds increases, the melting point of the fat decreases. Therefore, saturated fats are normally solids at room temperature, whereas unsaturated fats are liquids. Complete oxidation of 1 g of fat yields about 9 calories, whereas 1 g of carbohydrate yields about 4 calories.

18. **The correct answer is (C).** Messenger RNA transfers genetic information from the nucleus by forming a complex with the ribosomes (composed largely of ribosomal RNA) of the endoplasmic reticulum in the cytoplasm. Transfer RNA carries amino acids to the messenger RNA-ribosome complex during protein synthesis.

19. **The correct answer is (D).** Each mitotic division is a continuous process, with each stage merging imperceptibly into the next. For descriptive purposes, mitosis is divided into four successive stages: prophase, metaphase, anaphase, and telophase.

20. **The correct answer is (B).** Since biological membranes are primarily a sandwich composed of a bimolecular layer of lipid with a layer of protein on both the inner and outer surfaces, lipid-soluble compounds diffuse through it faster than water-soluble compounds. For water-

soluble compounds, the size of the molecule is the rate-limiting factor in diffusion.

21. **The correct answer is (D).** Passive diffusion of a substance requires no energy (ATP) and will therefore not be affected by a metabolic inhibitor (cyanide). Passive diffusion also transfers uncharged (more lipid-soluble) molecules from a higher to a lower concentration.

22. **The correct answer is (A).** A large sodium (Na^+) influx into the cell results in the resting potential (–50 mV) becoming more positive and thereby initiates the action potential. Potassium is already in very high concentration (~141 mEq/liter) intracellularly and will not enter the cell.

23. **The correct answer is (D).** A large efflux of potassium (K^+) out of the cell results in a fall in electrical potential within the cell. Potassium, in high concentration intracellularly, easily leaves the cell, whereas sodium, in high concentration extracellularly, will not diffuse out of the cell rapidly.

24. **The correct answer is (C).** The normal resting potential of –50 mV is established by the sodium-potassium pump of the cell, resulting in a high extracellular sodium concentration (~142 mEq/liter) and a high intracellular potassium concentration (A~141 mE~/liter). A negative resting potential is necessary to allow proper initiation of an action potential.

25. **The correct answer is (B).** Insulin is a hormone that decreases blood glucose levels by increasing glucose uptake and storage by the cells. Pepsin, trypsin, and lactase are enzymes necessary for the proper digestion of nutrients.

26. **The correct answer is (C).** The liver is the primary site of metabolism for the body and is responsible for detoxifying toxic agents in the blood. The lungs and kidneys both excrete these metabolized agents from the body. The pancreas does not directly metabolize toxic agents to any extent.

27. **The correct answer is (C).** The kidneys remove waste products from the body.

28. **The correct answer is (D).** All these processes are involved in the absorption of carbohydrates, amino acids, and fatty acids, as well as minerals and vitamins.

29. **The correct answer is (A).** Bile salts are necessary for the proper digestion of fats because they emulsify fat globules and render the end products of fat digestion soluble for more efficient absorption.

30. **The correct answer is (C).** Glucose, fructose, and galactose are all simple sugars derived from hydrolytic cleavage of polysaccharides and double sugars. These simple sugars are then readily absorbed from the digestive tract. Glycogen is the storage form of glucose in the different cells of the body.

31. **The correct answer is (A).** The brain does not store glucose as glycogen and must receive all its energy from glucose in the blood. Therefore, a rapid decrease in blood glucose immediately deprives the brain of the energy source it requires for normal function.

32. **The correct answer is (D).** Vitamin A, or retinol, is converted in the retina to retinal, a light-sensitive pigment, necessary for night vision.

33. **The correct answer is (B).** Both active transport and facilitated diffusion require carriers that combine with the transported substance. Passive diffusion involves the transfer of a substance from a region of higher concentration to one of lower concentration without a carrier.

34. **The correct answer is (B).** Saturation of the carrier with the transferring substance in active transport and facilitated diffusion will lead to saturation kinetics. In addition, phagocytosis also has a maximum rate of transfer. Passive diffusion does not have any of these restrictions and normally proceeds at a rate proportional to the amount of substance present for transfer.

35. **The correct answer is (C).** Mendel's first law, called the law of segregation, states that genes exist in individuals as pairs. The theory of recapitulation states that organisms tend to repeat, in the course of their evolutionary development, some of the corresponding stages of their evolutionary ancestors. Starling's law, also known as Starling's law of the heart, deals with regulation of the amount of blood pumped by the heart at a given time. The Watson-Crick model explains how the DNA molecule transfers information and undergoes replication.

36. **The correct answer is (D).** About 56 percent of the adult human body is water (H_2O), with the rest of the body being primarily composed of organic molecules containing carbon. Therefore, of the four stated elements, calcium would be the least abundant in the human body.

37. **The correct answer is (C).** Most species of animals and plants have chromosome numbers between 10 and 50. Humans have 46 chromosomes in each of their cells. Abnormalities in the chromosome number include Turner's syndrome (45 chromosomes) and Klinefelter's syndrome (47 chromosomes).

38. **The correct answer is (A).** O-negative blood, by definition, contains no A, B, or Rh agglutinogens that would cause a transfusion reaction and possibly death for a blood recipient. Therefore, O-negative blood can be given to any individuals of the four major blood types.

39. **The correct answer is (D).** Epinephrine is one of the neurotransmitters in the brain, especially in the thalamus and hypothalamus. Both norepinephrine and acetylcholine are transmitter substances known to be secreted by the autonomic nerves innervating smooth muscle. Cholecystokinin is a hormone secreted by the intestinal mucosa that causes specific contraction of the gallbladder.

40. **The correct answer is (D).** Neutrophils, monocytes, eosinophils, and basophils are white blood cells produced by the bone marrow along with red blood cells. Lymphocytes are white blood cells that are produced by lymphoid tissue.

41. **The correct answer is (A).** Actively acquired immunity depends on the production of specific proteins, antibodies, that are released into the blood and tissue fluids in response to some foreign protein (an antigen) or vaccine. On the other hand, passively acquired immunity is a result of the injection of antibodies that have been produced in another individual or species. Natural immunity protects humans from infectious diseases associated with animals, such as canine distemper. Cellular immunity deals with the recognition and destruction of foreign, genetically different cells and may be the cause of the rejection of transplanted organs.

42. **The correct answer is (C).** Glomerular filtration is the process by which the kidney removes most of the waste products from the blood by pure filtration through the glomerular membrane. Hydrogen ions undergo tubular secretion into the glomerular filtrate, whereas substances such as glucose, amino acids, and potassium ions are actively reabsorbed by the tubular membrane. Sublimation is a physical change from the solid directly to the gaseous state and does not apply to the kidney or any other organ.

43. The correct answer is (C). Stimulation of the sympathetic nervous system increases the heart rate, sweating, and blood pressure and dilates the pupils of the eyes. Stimulation of the parasympathetic nervous system produces opposite effects, that is, decreases the heart rate, sweating, and blood pressure, as well as constriction of the pupils.

44. The correct answer is (B). During heavy exercise, glycogen in the muscle breaks down to lactic acid faster than lactic acid can be oxidized, resulting in lactic acid accumulation.

45. The correct answer is (C). Meiosis occurs during the formation of eggs or sperm, where a pair of cell divisions result in gametes with only half the number of chromosomes (haploid) as the other cells of the body. When two gametes unite in fertilization, the fusion of their nuclei reconstitutes the diploid number of chromosomes.

46. The correct answer is (B). The physical appearance of any individual with respect to a given inherited trait is known as his or her phenotype. In contrast, an individual's genetic constitution, usually expressed in symbols, is called his or her genotype. Both recessive and heterozygous traits are related more to genotype rather than phenotype.

47. The correct answer is (A). Sickle-cell anemia is a condition where homozygous recessive genes are necessary for full development of the disease. If an individual has heterozygous recessive genes for the disease, that individual only shows sickle-cell trait, but not the fully developed disease. Both beriberi and pellagra are diseases associated with vitamin deficiencies. Hypertension is usually of unknown etiology.

48. The correct answer is (C). Intense exercise and training of an athlete can result in a decreased respiratory rate and an increase in the size in muscle fibers. However, there will be no increase in the number of muscle fibers, because this does not change after birth.

49. The correct answer is (D). Spermatogonia (diploid) grow into primary spermatocytes (diploid) and then secondary spermatocytes (diploid) after the first meiotic division. Secondary spermatocytes become spermatids (haploid) after the second meiotic division.

50. The correct answer is (A). An individual with type A-negative blood can receive blood from A-negative or O-negative donors. Rh-positive blood cannot be given, because a transfusion reaction would result. B- and AB-type bloods cannot be given for the same reason.

51. The correct answer is (D). The appendix, wisdom teeth, and coccygeal vertebrae (tail bone) serve no useful purpose in humans; however, the pupils of the eyes are necessary for sight.

52. The correct answer is (C). Graph C depicts a saturated reaction, as indicated by the initially straight lines for the product and substrate. The reaction proceeds to no substrate and all product, suggesting an irreversible reaction. Graph B indicates an unsaturated (curved lines) but irreversible (no substrate, all product after considerable time) reaction. Graph D represents an unsaturated reversible reaction, as shown by the initially curved line. This reaction also appears to be reversible, because the product and substrate appear to have reached an equilibrium. Thus, not all the substrate can be converted to product without some of the product reconverting to substrate.

53. The correct answer is (C). The transport of oxygen and carbon dioxide in the blood largely depends on the amount of hemoglobin present in the red blood cell. Whole blood carries approximately 20 ml of oxygen and 30–60 ml of carbon dioxide per 100 ml. Plasma water carries only about 0.2–0.3 ml of oxygen and carbon dioxide in each 100 ml. Plasma proteins carry essentially no oxygen.

54. **The correct answer is (A).** Breeding between closely related individuals, commonly referred to as inbreeding, increases the proportion of homozygous individuals in a population, promoting the occurrence of double recessive traits of congenital anomalies. Some genetic disorders, including muscular dystrophy and red-green color blindness, are sex-linked defective traits.

55. **The correct answer is (A).** Beneficial associations or interactions between two species of animals include commensalism, protocooperation, and mutualism. Negative interactions between two species include amensalism, parasitism, and predation.

56. **The correct answer is (D).** This question is similar to Question 52. Graph D shows unsaturated reaction characteristics (initially curved lines).

57. **The correct answer is (B).** Albumin (~5 g/100 ml of plasma) is the plasma protein most responsible for the osmotic pressure. Both fibrinogen and gammaglobulin are plasma proteins that contribute to the colloid osmotic pressure but to a considerably lesser degree. Hemoglobin is a red pigment responsible for the transport of oxygen and carbon dioxide in the blood.

58. **The correct answer is (C).** Only red blood cells carry hemoglobin, the substance responsible for oxygen and carbon dioxide transport.

59. **The correct answer is (D).** Plasma cells, derived from lymphocytes, produce and secrete antibodies. Thrombocytes, important in initiating the clotting of blood, are formed by the fragmentation of giant cells, megakaryocytes, in the red bone marrow. Neutrophils are important in taking up bacteria and dead tissue cells by phagocytosis.

60. **The correct answer is (A).** Cyanide is routinely employed as an inhibitor of enzymatic reactions. Therefore, treatment with cyanide will arrest the enzymatic reaction, and substrate will not be changed to product (Graph A).

61. **The correct answer is (C).** The hemoglobin in the red blood cell has a high capacity for binding both oxygen and carbon dioxide. A lack of hemoglobin (anemia) results in a decreased capacity for oxygen and carbon dioxide transport.

62. **The correct answer is (A).** Albumin (5 g/100 ml of plasma) is approximately 2.5 times more abundant than globulin (2 g/100 ml of plasma). Fibrinogen and immunoglobulins are present in small amounts compared to albumin.

63. **The correct answer is (D).** Whereas decreased oxygen delivery to tissues (or a low blood oxygen concentration) will increase the number of red blood cells, increased carbon dioxide concentration will not. Changes in the number of red blood cells appear to be associated with changes in blood oxygen tension rather than in blood carbon dioxide tension.

64. **The correct answer is (B).** Sweating, increases metabolism, and vasodilation of the blood vessels help transfer body heat to the surrounding environment. Increased muscle tone does not significantly increase heat loss.

65. **The correct answer is (C).** Urea and creatinine normally pass through the kidney in the glomerular filtrate. Conversely, normally all the glucose in the glomerular filtrate is actively reabsorbed by the kidney in the normal individual. Glucose can be found in the urine when the blood glucose concentration is abnor-

mally elevated (> 180 mg percent), as in uncontrolled diabetes.

66. **The correct answer is (D).** The reticular activating system is involved in the control of sleep, wakefulness, attentiveness, and behavior but does not actively participate in regulating the volume of body fluids. The baroreceptors and vasomotor center of the brain work together to increase the flow of blood to the glomeruli of the kidneys, resulting in increased glomerular filtration and formation of urine. The osmoreceptors control the amount of water reabsorbed from the tubular filtrate of the kidneys by the secretion of antidiuretic hormone.

67. **The correct answer is (C).** The axon and dendrites are components of the neuron. The dendrites constitute that part of the neuron specialized for receiving excitation, whereas the axon is the part specialized to distribute or conduct excitation away from the dendritic zone. Nerves are usually composed of collections of axons.

68. **The correct answer is (A).** The rate of conduction increases as the diameter of the axon increases because there is less resistance to the action potential. Thus, larger nerve fibers have a faster rate of conduction than smaller ones. Myelin sheaths usually increase the rate of conduction by insulating the action potential on the axon from the external environment, again decreasing resistance.

69. **The correct answer is (B).** The autonomic nervous system, composed of both sympathetic and parasympathetic nerves, is responsible for the involuntary activities of the body. Motor impulses reach the effector organ from the brain or spinal cord through a series of motor neurons comprising the corticospinal (pyramidal) and extracorticospinal (extrapyramidal).

70. **The correct answer is (D).** Thyroxine is an iodinated derivative of the amino acid tyrosine. Other hormones derived from amino acids include melatonin and epinephrine. Prostaglandins are derivatives of 20-carbon unsaturated fatty acids, whereas estradiol and testosterone are derived from cholesterol.

71. **The correct answer is (C).** A single muscle twitch is caused by an initiating action potential; however, there is a latent period after the generation of the action potential and initiation of the muscle twitch. After the latent period, the muscle contracts and then relaxes, followed by a refractory period in which the muscle will not respond to another action potential.

72. **The correct answer is (D).** The nervous system provides instantaneous control of a body function, whereas hormones usually take a relatively long time (hours or days) to regulate a body function.

73. **The correct answer is (A).** Progesterone is secreted by the corpus luteum and acts with estradiol to regulate the estrous and menstrual cycles. Vasopressin, secreted by the hypothalamus, stimulates the contraction of smooth muscles and has an antidiuretic action on kidney tubules. Aldosterone regulates metabolism of sodium and potassium and is secreted by the adrenal cortex.

74. **The correct answer is (C).** The rods of the retina are responsible for peripheral, achromatic, and poor detail visions. Central, color, and detail visions are a function of the cones of the retina.

75. **The correct answer is (A).** The rate of lymph flow is much slower (~100 ml/hr.) than blood flow (~5 liter/min.) in humans and most animal species.

Quantitative Ability

1.	C	21.	C	41.	A	61.	C	81.	C
2.	B	22.	C	42.	D	62.	A	82.	D
3.	A	23.	B	43.	B	63.	C	83.	A
4.	D	24.	D	44.	D	64.	C	84.	B
5.	C	25.	C	45.	D	65.	C	85.	C
6.	C	26.	C	46.	B	66.	B	86.	D
7.	B	27.	C	47.	C	67.	B	87.	A
8.	C	28.	B	48.	C	68.	C	88.	A
9.	C	29.	A	49.	A	69.	C	89.	A
10.	C	30.	C	50.	A	70.	A	90.	B
11.	B	31.	C	51.	A	71.	D	91.	D
12.	D	32.	B	52.	B	72.	D	92.	A
13.	C	33.	C	53.	B	73.	A	93.	B
14.	D	34.	B	54.	A	74.	C	94.	D
15.	D	35.	D	55.	D	75.	A	95.	D
16.	A	36.	B	56.	D	76.	B	96.	A
17.	C	37.	A	57.	A	77.	B	97.	B
18.	D	38.	A	58.	D	78.	D	98.	D
19.	B	39.	D	59.	B	79.	A	99.	C
20.	A	40.	B	60.	B	80.	C	100.	A

1. **The correct answer is (C).** To add or subtract fractions, convert to equivalent fractions with the same least common denominator (LCD):

$$\frac{3}{8}+\frac{4}{5}=\frac{3\times 5}{8\times 5}+\frac{4\times 8}{5\times 8}$$
$$=\frac{15}{40}+\frac{32}{40}$$
$$=\frac{47}{40}$$
$$=1\frac{7}{40}$$

2. **The correct answer is (B).** To add or subtract arithmetic fractions and decimal fractions, convert to a common base:

$$0.25+\frac{15}{16}=\frac{4}{16}+\frac{15}{16}$$
$$=\frac{19}{16}$$
$$=1\frac{3}{16}$$

or

$$0.25+\frac{15}{16}=0.25+0.9375$$
$$=1.1875$$

3. **The correct answer is (A).** The following relations may be used when dealing with scientific notation:

$$10^0 = 1$$
$$10^{-A} = \frac{1}{10^A}$$
$$10^{A+B} = 10^A \times 10^B$$
$$\frac{10^A}{10^B} = 10^{A-B}$$
$$\left(10^A\right)^B = 10^{AB}$$

Because
$$1.30 = 1.30 \times 10^0$$
and
$$236 = 2.36 \times 10^2$$
we have
$$(1.30 \times 10^0) \times (2.36 \times 10^2) = 3.068 \times 10^{0+2}$$
$$= 3.068 \times 10^2$$

4. **The correct answer is (D).** The log of a product equals the sum of the logs of the component numbers:

$$\log(50 \times 2) = \log 50 + \log 2 = \log 2 + \log 50$$

5. **The correct answer is (C).** The logs of multiples of 10, for example, 1, 10, 0.1, are integers:

$10^2 = 100$	$\log 100 = 2$
$10^1 = 10$	$\log 10 = 1$
$10^0 = 1$	$\log 1 = 0$
$10^{-1} = 0.1$	$\log 0.1 = -1$
$10^{-2} = 0.01$	$\log 0.01 = -2$
$10^{-3} = 0.001$	$\log 0.001 = -3$

6. **The correct answer is (C).** The root of a power is found by dividing the exponent of the power of the index of the root (see the law of exponents in Answer 19):

$$\sqrt[3]{8}$$

8 is the power

1 is the exponent

3 is the root

$$= 8^{\frac{1}{3}}$$

7. **The correct answer is (B).** The log of a number is the exponent of the power to which a given base must be raised to equal that number; that is, if:

$$y = a^x$$
then
$$\log_a y = x$$
Therefore,
$$\log_{10} 1,000 = 3$$
or base 10 raised to the third power equals 1,000.

8. **The correct answer is (C).** When adding or subtracting in scientific notation, convert to the same exponent, then add the products; the exponent will remain constant:

$$1 \times 10^{-2} = 0.01 \times 10^0$$
and
$$2.3 \times 10^1 = 23 \times 10^0$$
So,
$$(0.01 \times 10^0) + (23 \times 10^0) = 23.01 \times 10^0$$
$$= 23.01$$

9. **The correct answer is (C).** Percent, written as %, means per hundred. It is a type of ratio and thus has no units. To express a fraction as a percentage, set 100 as the denominator and multiply by 100%:

$$\frac{3}{16} \times 100\% = 0.1875 \times 100\%$$
$$= 18.75\%$$

10. **The correct answer is (C).** Weight-per-volume measurements are often expressed as percentages. To calculate the percent weight per volume, convert the fraction to a percentage, that is, with a denominator of 100, times 100%:

$$\frac{2.3\text{ g}}{10\text{ ml}} = \frac{23\text{ g}}{100\text{ ml}}$$
and
$$\frac{23\text{ g}}{100\text{ ml}} \times 100\% = 23\%\frac{\text{wt}}{\text{vol}}$$

11. **The correct answer is (B).** This problem involves the use of two ratios set equal to each other to form an equation known as a proportion. To solve a proportion, only one number may be unknown, which will be called x. To solve, rearrange the equation such that x remains alone. Given $A:B = C:D$, the following rules may be used:

1. The product of the means equals the product of the extremes: $B \times C = A \times D$.

2. The product of the means divided by one extreme gives the other extreme:
$$\frac{BC}{A} = D$$

3. The product of the extremes divided by one mean gives the other mean:
$$\frac{AD}{B} = C$$

Therefore,

$$4\% \text{ solution} = \frac{4 \text{ g}}{100 \text{ ml}}$$

(as explained in Answer 10) and

x = number of liters in which 24 g will be dissolved.

(Note: 1,000 ml. = 1 liter.)

Since

$$4 \text{ g} : 100 \text{ ml.} :: 24 \text{ g} : x \text{ ml.}$$

then

$$\frac{4 \text{ g}}{100 \text{ ml}} = \frac{24 \text{ g}}{x}$$
$$x = \frac{24 \text{ g} \times 100 \text{ ml}}{4 \text{ g}}$$
$$= 600 \text{ ml or 0.6 liter}$$

12. **The correct answer is (D).** This problem is similar to that of Question 11 because a proportionality is needed to solve the problem. First determine the total number of grams of NaCl that will be used to make the 0.9% solution:

$$18\% = \frac{18 \text{ g}}{100 \text{ ml}} \times 1,000 \text{ ml}$$
$$= 180 \text{ g}$$

This quantity will be diluted with the final total volume, the unknown x, which should result in a 0.9% solution:

$$0.9\% = \frac{0.9 \text{ g}}{100 \text{ ml}}$$

and

$$\frac{0.9 \text{ g}}{100 \text{ ml}} = \frac{180 \text{ g}}{x \text{ ml}}$$

So

$$x \text{ ml} = \frac{180 \text{ g} \times 100 \text{ ml}}{0.9 \text{ g}}$$
$$= 20,000 \text{ ml}$$
$$= 20 \text{ liters}$$

13. **The correct answer is (C).** When one mixes different strengths, the units and types of percent (wt/wt, wt/vol, vol/vol) must be kept constant. Determine the total amount of ethanol in all solutions and the total amount of solution, assuming additivity of volumes on mixing. Then, convert to the desired final ration:

$$25\% \times 5,000 \text{ ml} = 1,250 \text{ ml}$$
$$50\% \times 2,000 \text{ ml} = 1,000 \text{ ml}$$
$$10\% \times 500 \text{ ml} = 50 \text{ ml ethanol}$$

So,

$$\frac{1,250 + 1,000 + 50}{5,000 + 2,000 + 50} =$$
$$\frac{2,300 \text{ ml of ethanol}}{7,500 \text{ ml of solution}} = 0.3067 \cong 30.7\%$$

14. **The correct answer is (D).** The laws of logarithms are derived from the laws of exponents (see Answer 19). The most commonly used base is 10, although any base may be used.

$$\log (ab) = \log a + \log b$$

$$\log \left(\frac{a}{b}\right) = \log a - \log b$$

$$\log a^n = n \times \log a$$

$$\log a^{\frac{1}{n}} = \log \sqrt[n]{a} = \left(\frac{1}{n}\right)\log a$$

Therefore,

$$\log \sqrt{25} = \frac{1}{2}\log\ 25 = \frac{(\log\ 25)}{2}$$
$$= \log\ 25^{\frac{1}{2}}$$
$$= \log\ 5$$

15. **The correct answer is (D).** From previous answers:

$$\log a^n = n \times \log a$$

$$\log 25^2 = 2 \times \log 25$$

16. **The correct answer is (A).** This problem involves ratios. First convert the common units:

$$1\ \text{kg} = 1{,}000\ \text{g}$$

Then set up the proportionality:

$$\frac{1\ \text{kg}}{2.2\ \text{lb}} = \frac{x}{1\ \text{lb}}$$
$$\frac{1{,}000 \times (1\ \text{lb})}{2.2\ \text{lb}} = x$$
$$454.5\ \text{g} = x$$

17. **The correct answer is (C).** Whenever mathematical procedures are used, all the units must be the same.

Therefore,

$$1\ \text{liter} = 1{,}000\ \text{ml}$$

and

$$1{,}000\ \text{ml} - 283\ \text{ml} = 717\ \text{ml}$$

18. **The correct answer is (D).** (See Answers 11 and 16.)

Because 1 g = 1,000 mg

we have

$$\frac{15.43\ \text{grains}}{1{,}000\ \text{mg}} = \frac{1\ \text{grain}}{x\ \text{mg}}$$
$$x\ \text{mg} = \frac{1\ \text{grain} \times 1{,}000\ \text{mg}}{15.43\ \text{grains}}$$
$$x = 64.81\ \text{mg}$$

19. **The correct answer is (B).** First simplify the numbers (see Answer 6); then use the law of exponents:

1. The product of two or more powers of the *same base* is the base with an exponent equal to the *sum of all the exponents*:
$$4^3 \times 4^{10} = 4^{10+3} = 4^{13}$$

2. The quotient of two powers with the *same base* is the base with an exponent equal to the *exponent of the numerator minus that of the denominator*:
$$\frac{3^8}{3^2} = 3^{8-2} = 3^6$$

3. The power of a power is found by *multiplying the exponents*:
$$(2^4)^3 = 2^{4\times3} = 2^{12}$$

4. The power of a product equals the *product of the powers* of the factors:
$$(2 \times 3 \times 4)^2 = 2^2 \times 3^2 \times 4^2$$

5. The root of a power is found by *dividing the exponent of the power by the index of the root*:
$$\sqrt[3]{8^6} = 8^{\frac{6}{3}} = 8^2$$

6. The power of a fraction equals the *power of the numerator divided by the power of the denominator*:
$$\left(\frac{2}{3}\right)^2 = \frac{2^2}{3^2}$$

7. A number with a *negative* exponent equals 1 divided by the number with a positive exponent:
$$12^{-2} = \frac{1}{12^2}$$

8. Any number other than 0 with exponent 0 equals 1:
$$10^0 = 1, \; 4^0 = 1, \; 1^0 = 1$$

Therefore, for Question 19, we have
$\sqrt[3]{3^6} = 3^{\frac{6}{3}} = 3^2$ and $\sqrt{2^2} = 2^{\frac{2}{2}} = 2^1 = 2$ so,

$$3^2 + 2 = (3 \times 3) + 2$$

$$3^2 + 2 = 11$$

20. **The correct answer is (A).** Making the appropriate conversion to the least common denominator, we have:

$$\left(\frac{2}{3}\right)^2 + 2^{-3} = \frac{2^2}{3^2} + \frac{1}{2^3}$$
$$= \frac{4}{9} + \frac{1}{8}$$
$$= \frac{4 \times 8}{9 \times 8} + \frac{1 \times 9}{8 \times 9}$$
$$= \frac{32}{72} + \frac{9}{72}$$
$$= \frac{41}{72}$$

21. **The correct answer is (C).**

$$10^0 = 1$$
$$10^1 = 10$$
$$\underline{10^{-1} = 0.1}$$
$$11.1$$

22. **The correct answer is (C).** In problems involving formulas, rearrange the formula until the unknown term is expressed by all the other terms. Therefore, if the temperature in degrees centigrade is unknown, rearrange the formula as follows:

$$9(x°C) = 5(y°F) - 160$$
$$x°C = \frac{5}{9}(y°F) - \frac{160}{9}$$
$$= \frac{5 \times 79}{9} - 17.78$$
$$= 26.1$$

23. **The correct answer is (B).** Rearrange to solve for the temperature in degrees Fahrenheit.

$$
\begin{aligned}
9(x°C) &= 5(y°F) - 160 \\
5(y°F) &= 9(x°C) + 160 \\
y°F &= \frac{9}{5}(x°C) + \frac{160}{5} \\
&= \frac{9° \times (-10°)}{5°} + 32° \\
&= -18° + 32° \\
&= 14°F
\end{aligned}
$$

24. **The correct answer is (D).** This problem may be approached by determining the respective temperatures in degrees centigrade and then computing the difference.

    From
    $$x°C = \frac{5(y°F) - 160}{9}$$
    we have
    $$x°C = \frac{5(72) - 160}{9}, \quad x'°C = \frac{5(65) - 160}{9}$$
    $$x°C = 22.22, \quad\quad x'°C \cong 18.33$$
    So,
    $$22.22 - 18.33 \cong 3.88 \quad\quad 3.9°C$$

    Alternately, because 1°F is $\frac{9}{5}$ of a degree on the centigrade scale, the problem may be solved by multiplying the differences in degrees Fahrenheit by $\frac{5}{9}$.

    $$72°F - 65°F = 7°F$$

    $$7°F \times \frac{5}{9} = \frac{35}{9} = 3.88°C$$

    You cannot directly substitute the 7°F into the temperature conversion equation as originally given, since that equation converts the 7°F to the corresponding temperature in degrees centigrade. That is, 7°F equals –13.8°C.

25. **The correct answer is (C).** This is a proportionality problem. Assume a weight-volume relationship:
    $$1 : 10,000 :: x : 200 :$$

    $$\frac{1\text{ g}}{10,000\text{ ml}} = \frac{x\text{ g}}{200\text{ ml}}$$
    $$x\text{ g} = \frac{(1\text{ g}) \times (200\text{ ml})}{10,000\text{ ml}}$$
    $$= 0.02\text{ g}$$

26. **The correct answer is (C).** When x is known, y may be found by drawing a line up from the x-axis, parallel to the y-axis, until the line of the graph is intersected. A line is then drawn from this point perpendicular to the y-axis until it is intersected. This is the value of y for a given x.

27. **The correct answer is (C).** The rate of drug disappearance is the change in y (mg drug/ml plasma) over a range of x (time). This is equal to the slope:
    $$\frac{y_2 - y_1}{x_2 - x_1} = m$$
    Therefore, to determine the rate (slope), any two y-values and corresponding x-values are needed. For example,

    $$\text{time}_1 = 0\text{ min.}, \quad y_1 = \frac{\text{mg drug}}{\text{mg plasma}} = 4$$

    $$\text{time}_2 = 80\text{ min.}, \quad y_2 = \frac{\text{mg drug}}{\text{mg plasma}} = 2$$

    Then,
    $$\text{rate} = \frac{2 - 4}{80 - 0} = \frac{-2}{80} = \frac{-1}{40}$$
    and
    $$\frac{-1}{40} = \frac{-1\text{ mg/ml plasma}}{40\text{ min.}}$$
    $$= -1.5\text{ mg/ml plasma per hour}$$

    Note: The negative sign indicates a decline, or falling y values, for increasing x values.

28. **The correct answer is (B).** To predict a y value for a given x, the slope m and the y-intercept b must be known so we can solve $y = mx + b$. From Answer 27:
    $$m = \frac{-1.5\text{ mg/ml plasma}}{1\text{ hr.}}$$
    and
    $$b = 4\text{ mg/ml plasma}$$
    $$x = 2\text{ hrs.}$$
    So,
    $$y = (-1.5\text{ mg/ml per hour}) \times (2\text{ hrs.}) + 4\text{ mg/ml}$$
    $$= -3\text{ mg/ml} + 4\text{ mg/ml}$$
    $$= 1\text{ mg/ml}$$

    Remember to include the negative sign in the slope.

29. **The correct answer is (A).** In this problem, the y-intercept has been changed to 8 mg/ml. and the time to 80 min. (1.33 hrs.). The problem is then solved as in Answer 28:

$y = mx + b$

$= (-1.5 \text{ mg/ml per hour}) \times (1.33 \text{ hrs.}) + 8 \text{ mg/hr.}$

$= -1.995 + 8$

$\cong 6 \text{ mg/ml.}$

30. **The correct answer is (C).** This problem requires finding the value of x (time) when y (concentration) is zero. Again,

y is $mx + b$

$0 = (-1.5 \text{ mg/ml per hour})x + 4 \text{ mg/ml}$

$\dfrac{-4 \text{ mg/ml}}{-1.5 \text{ mg/ml per hour}} = x$

$2.66 \text{ hrs.} = x$

$160 \text{ min.} = x$

31. **The correct answer is (C).** An integer is any of the natural numbers, the negatives of the numbers and zero. To find the values for the inequalities, solve each of the inequalities separately; then delete all values not satisfying both:

$4 < 3x - 2 \le 10$	$3x - 2 \le 10$
$4 < 3x - 2$	$3x \le 10 + 2$
$4 + 2 < 3x$	$3x \le 12$
$\dfrac{6}{3} < x$	$x \le 4$
$2 < x$	

Therefore, all values greater than 2 may be accepted: 3, 4, 5, ..., n

Therefore, all values less than or equal to 4 will be accepted: 4, 3, 2, 1, 0, –1, –2, ..., –n

Integer values common to both inequalities are 3 and 4.

32. **The correct answer is (B).**

$\dfrac{7}{x} > 2, \qquad x \ne 0$

$7 > 2x$

$\dfrac{7}{2} > x$

$3.5 > x$

x must be less than 3.5, or 3, 2, 1, 0, –1, –2..., but x cannot be 0; therefore, 3, 2, and 1 are common to both equations.

33. **The correct answer is (C).** The absolute value $|x|$ removes the sign of the number enclosed after all arithmetic functions enclosed have been completed, or $|-x| = x$.

Therefore,

$|-5| - |-2| = 5 - 2 = 3$

34. **The correct answer is (B).**

$|8| - |14| = 8 - 14 = -6$

35. **The correct answer is (D).**

$|5x + 4| = -3$

This problem cannot be solved, because there is no term whose absolute value will yield a negative result.

36. **The correct answer is (B).** Because the figure is a cube, D is the hypotenuse of a right triangle with equal sides. From the Pythagorean theorem, we have hypotenuse^2 = side^2 + side^2.

$x^2 = 2^2 + 2^2$

$x^2 = 4 + 4$

$x^2 = 8$

$x = \sqrt{8}$

37. The correct answer is (A). In this example, lines *C*, *D*, and *E* form a right triangle with base *D* and side *C* (or base *C* and side *D*). If *C* is 2 in. (given condition) and *D*, from the previous example, is $\sqrt{8}$ in., then $\frac{1}{2}\sqrt{8}$ (2) = $\sqrt{8}$ in.² (The area of a triangle is equal to $\frac{1}{2}$ base × height.) *E* could also serve as a base, except, because *E* was unknown, it was easier to work with the sides already known.

38. The correct answer is (A). A cube has six faces: top, bottom, and four sides. If each face has a surface area of 2 × 2 in.², then the total area is

$$\frac{(2 \text{ in.} \times 2 \text{ in.})}{\text{face}} \times 6 \text{ faces} = 24 \text{ in.}^2$$

39. The correct answer is (D). The subset of *A or B* includes all subsets for *A* (1, 2) plus all subsets of *B* (2, 3, 4); that is, all cases in which the condition of *A or B* has been met will be accepted (1, 2, 3, 4).

40. The correct answer is (B). A subset *A and B* includes all cases in which both the conditions of subset *A* and subset *B* must be met (2 only).

41. The correct answer is (A). The subset *A or C* includes all cases satisfying the conditions of subset *A* (1, 2) plus those satisfying the conditions of *C* (4, 5). However, any cases also included in *B* must be excluded (2, 3, or 4), because the subset we are looking for is *A or C, but not B*. Therefore, only subsets 1 and 5 may be accepted.

42. The correct answer is (D). The subset "only" means that any other conditions being met must be excluded. Therefore, although *B* is composed of 2, 3, and 4, only 3 may be accepted, because 2 is also a subset of *A* and 4 is also a subset of *C*.

43. The correct answer is (B).

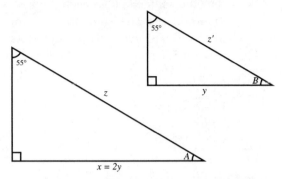

The ratio of the areas of similar triangles is equal to the square of the ratio of corresponding sides. Therefore, when *x* = 2*y*, the ratio of the sides is $\frac{2}{1} : \frac{x}{y}$ because *x* is twice the value of *y*. The ratio of the areas is then $\left(\frac{2}{1}\right)^2$ or $\frac{4}{1}$ or 4:1.

44. The correct answer is (D). The sum of all angles in a triangle is 180°. If one angle is 55° and a right angle is 90°, then angle *A* is 180° − 55° − 90° = 35°.

45. The correct answer is (D). Since the two triangles are similar, if *x* = 3*y*, then:

z = 3*z*′, or

$$z' = \frac{z}{3} = \frac{5}{3} = 1\frac{2}{3}$$

46. The correct answer is (B). The value of a bar graph is determined by drawing a line perpendicular to the *y*-axis from the top of the graph. The point of interception is the *y*-value of that bar.

Therefore, only *B* and *C* have 90% or more of the active ingredient as declared by the manufacturer.

47. The correct answer is (C). If sample B was 100% of claim and C was 120%, then the amount of drug present is:

100% × 200 mg = 1 × 200 = 200 mg

120% × 200 mg = 1.2 × 200 = 240 mg

48. The correct answer is (C). The mean is the sum of all values divided by the number of samples:

$\overline{X} = \frac{1}{N} \Sigma\, x$ when N is the number of samples and x is the value of each sample. From the bar graph, the following values were obtained:

1 score of 20	20 = (1 × 20)
1 score of 30	30 = (1 × 30)
1 score of 40	40 = (1 × 40)
1 score of 100	100 = (1 × 100)
2 scores of 50	100 = (2 × 50)
2 scores of 90	180 = (2 × 90)
3 scores of 60	180 = (3 × 60)
4 scores of 80	320 = (4 × 80)
5 scores of 70	350 = (5 × 70)

$N = 20 = $ number of samples

Σ of all values = 1,320

$\frac{1}{N} \Sigma\, x = \frac{1,320}{20} = 66 = $ mean

49. The correct answer is (A). The *modal score* is the most frequently occurring score. As 5 students scored 70% and no other score occurred as frequently, 70% is the modal score.

50. The correct answer is (A). The *median* is the term that is larger than or equal to half the terms and equal to or smaller than the other half of them. In this example, there are scores for a total of 20 students. As there are an even number of terms, there exists no actual median; that is, no term larger than exactly half of the terms and smaller than the other half. However, now it is pos-

sible to find two middle terms, and the median is defined as the mean of these two middle terms. In this example, if the scores are ranked in ascending order, the two middle scores are 70 and 70:

1.	20	6.	60	*11.	70	16.	80
2.	30	7.	60	12.	70	17.	80
3.	40	8.	60	13.	70	18.	90
4.	50	9.	70	14.	80	19.	90
5.	50	*10.	70	15.	80	20.	100

*As rank position, 10 and 11 are in the middle; that is, 70 is larger than or equal to half of the terms and equal to or smaller than half, and because 70 is the mean of 70 and 70, the median is 70.

51. The correct answer is (A). This is a proportionality problem:

$0.625\text{ g} : 50 :: 31.25\text{ g} : x$

$$\frac{0.625}{50} = \frac{31.25}{x}$$

$$x \text{ tablets} = \frac{31.25\text{ g} \times 50 \text{ tablets}}{0.625\text{ g}}$$

$$= 2{,}500 \text{ tablets}$$

52. The correct answer is (B). Assuming that the dose should be directly related to body weight, we set up a proportion:

$$\frac{70\ \mu g}{150\ \text{lb}} = \frac{x\ \mu g}{44\ \text{lb}}$$

$$x\ \mu g = \frac{70\ \mu g \times 44\ \text{lb}}{150\ \text{lb}}$$

$$x = 20.53\ \mu g \cong 20\ \mu g$$

53. The correct answer is (B). To solve for changes in y relative to x, rearrange the equation in terms of y:

$$x = \frac{1}{y}$$

$$y = \frac{1}{x}$$

Then, substitute in the change:

$$y = \frac{1}{x(2)} = \left(\frac{1}{x}\right) \times \frac{1}{2}$$

Therefore, it can be seen that when x increases by a factor of 2, y is halved.

54. **The correct answer is (A).** Rearrange the equation in terms of y (see Answer 53):

$$x = 2y$$

$$y = \frac{x}{2}$$

Increase x by a factor of 2:

$$y = \frac{x \times 2}{2}$$

y has increased by a factor of 2.

55. **The correct answer is (D).** This is a simple fraction problem. The question is: how many times does 16 go into 24?

$$\frac{24 \text{ g}}{16} = 1.5 \text{ g} = 1,500 \text{ mg}$$

56. **The correct answer is (D).** Determine the weight that represents a 10% error. The range of acceptable weights would be all the tablet weights that are within 150 g ± the 10% error:

$$150 \text{ g} \times \frac{10\%}{100\%} = 15 \text{ g}$$

$$150 \text{ g} - 15 \text{ g} = 135 \text{ g}$$

$$150 \text{ g} + 15 \text{ g} = 165 \text{ g}$$

So, the range is 135–165 g.

57. **The correct answer is (A).** A percentage is the amount per hundred. A proportion should then be set up to find how much iron is in 100 mg of ferrous sulfate, knowing the ratio of 65 mg/325 mg, iron to ferrous sulfate:

$$\frac{x}{100\%} = \frac{65 \text{ mg of iron}}{325 \text{ mg of ferrous sulfate}}$$

$$\frac{65 \text{ mg}}{325 \text{ mg}} \times 100\% = 20\%$$

58. **The correct answer is (D).** Set up a proportion with x representing the number of milligrams of compound in a liter (remember, 1 liter equals 1,000 ml):

$$\frac{x \text{ mg}}{1,000 \text{ ml}} = \frac{50 \text{ mg}}{\text{ml}}$$

$$x \text{ mg} = \frac{50 \text{ mg} \times 1,000 \text{ ml}}{\text{ml}}$$

$$= 50,000 \text{ mg}$$

As 1,000 mg are in 1 g,

$$\frac{50,000 \text{ g}}{1,000 \text{ mg/1 g}} = 50 \text{ g}$$

59. **The correct answer is (B).** If 5 ml is the smallest unit marked, then all errors are related to this unit and all readings would be rounded off to multiples of that unit; 5 ml represents the potential error. In this problem, the potential error is also the percentage error of a measured volume (x ml):

$$\frac{5 \text{ ml}}{x \text{ ml}} \times 100\% = \text{ percentage error}$$

$$\frac{500\%}{x \text{ ml}} = 10\%$$

$$x \text{ ml} = \frac{500\%}{10\%}$$

$$x = 50 \text{ ml}$$

60. **The correct answer is (B).** The average is analogous to the mean:

$$\frac{1}{N} \Sigma \text{ values} = \text{average}$$

$$\frac{61 + 50 + 100 + 50}{1 + 1 + 1 + 1} = 65.25 = 65$$

61. **The correct answer is (C).** The equation for a straight line is $y = mx + b$, where b is the y-intercept and m is the slope.

Thus:

$$y = mx + b$$

$$y = -0.118x + 8.5$$

62. **The correct answer is (A).** Rearrange the equation of the line to isolate x; then, substitute the value of the y-intercept:

$$y = -0.118x + 8.5$$

$$y - 8.5 = -0.118x$$

$$\left[\frac{y - 8.5}{-0.118}\right] = x$$

$$\left[\frac{6 - 8.5}{-0.118}\right] = x$$

$$21 = x$$

63. **The correct answer is (C).** The value of y, when x is zero, is 8.5. For all other values of x, solve for y by substituting into the equation of the line.

64. **The correct answer is (C).** The volume of the cylinder is $\pi r^2 h$, where h (height) is 10 and r (radius) is 2:

$$\text{volume} = \pi r^2 h$$

$$= (3.14)(2^2)(10)$$

$$= 125.6 \text{ units}^3$$

$$= 126 \text{ units}^3$$

65. **The correct answer is (C).** The lateral surface area is the circumference of the end, $2\pi r$, times the height:

$$\text{Lateral surface} = (2\pi r)(h)$$

$$= (2)(3.14)(2)(10)$$

$$= 125.6$$

$$= 126 \text{ units}^2$$

66. **The correct answer is (B).** The total area is the area of the lateral surface plus the areas of both ends:

$$\text{area of circle} = \pi r^2$$

$$\text{lateral surface} = 2\pi r h$$

$$\text{total area} = (2)(\pi r^2) + (2\pi r h)$$

$$= 2\pi r\,(r + h)$$

$$= (2)(3.14)(2)(2 + 10)$$

$$= 150.7$$

$$= 151 \text{ units}^2$$

67. **The correct answer is (B).** The area of a trapezoid is $\frac{1}{2}(h)(a + b)$:

$$\frac{1}{2}(1)(4 + 2) = \text{area}$$

$$3 \text{ units}^2 = \text{area}$$

68. **The correct answer is (C).** The area of a parallelogram is determined by $h \times b$:

$$(2)(5) = \text{area}$$

$$10 \text{ units}^2 = \text{area}$$

69. **The correct answer is (C).** To solve simultaneous equations, isolate the term in the first equation, which will be subsequently inserted into the second equation. In this case, y will be expressed in terms of x and b. The a term is common to both; therefore, rearrange the x equation to isolate a:

$$x = 3b + a$$

$$a = x - 3b$$

Then, substitute into the y equation:

$$y = 3a + b = 3(x - 3b) + b$$

$$= 3x - 9b + b = 3x - 8b$$

70. **The correct answer is (A).** The slope of a line (I) is the change in y versus the change in x (x versus y). The ordinate (y-value) intercept is given by c. The abscissa (x-value) intercept occurs when y equals zero or $0 = mx + c$, $x = \frac{-c}{m}$.

71. **The correct answer is (D).** When one divides ratios with the same denominator, the denominators may be factored out and only the numerators divided. It may be viewed in any of the following fashions:

$$\frac{7 \div 3}{21 \div 3} = \frac{7}{21} = \frac{1}{3} = 0.33$$

$$7 : 3 :: 21 : 3 \rightarrow \frac{7}{21} = \frac{1}{3} = 0.33$$

$$\frac{7}{\cancel{3}} \div \frac{21}{\cancel{3}} = \frac{7}{21} = \frac{1}{3} = 0.33$$

72. The correct answer is (D). To reduce a fraction, first determine what roots of the numerator are common in the denominator:

$$\frac{72}{2,880} = \frac{72}{72 \times 40} \text{ or } \frac{2 \times 2 \times 2 \times 3 \times 3}{2 \times 2 \times 2 \times 2 \times 2 \times 2 \times 2 \times 3 \times 3 \times 5}$$

$$= \frac{1}{2 \times 2 \times 2 \times 5}$$

$$= \frac{1}{40}$$

73. The correct answer is (A). Set up the proportion:

$$\frac{0.25 \text{ mg}}{\text{tablet}} = \frac{7.5 \text{ mg}}{x \text{ tablets}}$$

$$x = \frac{7.5 \text{ mg} \times 1 \text{ tablet}}{0.25 \text{ mg}}$$

$$x = 30$$

74. The correct answer is (C). Convert all the fractions to decimals; then, add all values:

$$\frac{3}{4} = \frac{x}{1.00} \qquad \frac{2}{5} = \frac{x}{1.00}$$

$$x = \frac{3 \times 1.00}{4} \qquad x = \frac{2 \times 1.00}{5}$$

$$x = 0.75 \qquad x = 0.40$$

$\frac{3}{4}$ mg $+ 0.25$ mg $+ \frac{2}{5}$ mg $+ 2.75$ mg $= x$ mg

$$0.75 + 0.25 + 0.40 + 2.75 = 4.15 \text{ mg}$$

75. The correct answer is (A). To add, convert all numbers to common units. In this case, grams (g) is the base unit:

$$1,000 \text{ mg} = 1 \text{ g}$$

$$1 \text{ kg} = 1,000 \text{ g}$$

Therefore,

$$\frac{0.75 \text{ mg}}{x \text{ g}} = \frac{1,000 \text{ mg}}{1 \text{ g}}$$

$$x \text{ g} = 0.00075 \text{ g}$$

$$\frac{0.5 \text{ kg}}{x \text{ g}} = \frac{1 \text{ kg}}{1,000 \text{ g}}$$

$$x \text{ g} = 500 \text{ g}$$

$$0.75 \text{ mg} + 50 \text{ g} + 0.5 \text{ kg} - x \text{ g}$$

$$0.00075 \text{ g} + 50 \text{ g} + 500 \text{ g} = 550.00075 \text{ g}$$

76. The correct answer is (B). Express $3\frac{1}{8}$ as a fraction:

$$\frac{3 \times 8}{8} + \frac{1}{8} = \frac{25}{8}$$

Then, convert the fraction so that it has a denominator common to those of the possible answers. Those values with a denominator of 36 may automatically be discarded, as 8 is not a factor of 36 (i.e., 36 cannot be divided by 8 to yield a whole number). Therefore, only denominators of 32 need be considered:

$$\frac{25 \times 4}{8 \times 4} = \frac{100}{32}$$

77. The correct answer is (B). First determine how many milligrams are being considered; then convert to grains by proportionalities:

$$\frac{10\%}{100\%} \times 360 = 36 \text{ mg}$$

$$\frac{1 \text{ grain}}{60 \text{ mg}} = \frac{x \text{ grain}}{36 \text{ mg}}$$

$$x \text{ grains} = 0.6 \text{ grain}$$

78. The correct answer is (D). Both quantities must first be converted to similar denominators; then, they can be simplified and added:

$$\frac{2\sqrt{36} \times 3\sqrt{7}}{3\sqrt{7}} + \frac{4\sqrt{28}}{3\sqrt{7}} = \frac{(2\sqrt{6 \times 6} \times 3\sqrt{7})}{3\sqrt{7}} + \frac{4\sqrt{2 \times 2 \times 7}}{3\sqrt{7}}$$

$$= \frac{(2 \times 6) \times (3\sqrt{7}) + 4\sqrt{2 \times 2} \times \sqrt{7}}{3\sqrt{7}}$$

$$= \frac{36 + 8}{3}$$

$$= 14\frac{2}{3}$$

79. The correct answer is (A). This is a simple substitution problem. If A were equal to x, then $1 + A$ would equal $1 + x$. The value of A does not change the mathematical principle. Therefore, when:

$$A = e^a$$

we have

$$1 + A = 1 + e^a$$

80. The correct answer is (C). Any number to the power of zero is 1:

$$7.7 \times 10^0 = 7.7 \times 1 = 7.7$$

81. The correct answer is (C). 1,000,000 expressed in base 10 is 1×10^6. Using the law of exponents (see Answer 19), we have:

$$1 \times 10^3 \times 10^3 = 1 \times 10^{3+3}$$
$$= 1 \times 10^6$$

82. The correct answer is (D). Using the law of exponents (see Answer 19), we see that $\sqrt{144 \times 10^4}$ may be broken down as follows:

$$\sqrt{144 \times 10^4} = \sqrt{144} \times \sqrt{10^4}$$
$$= \sqrt{12 \times 12} \times \sqrt{10^2 \times 10^2}$$
$$= 12 \times 10^2$$
$$= 1,200$$

83. The correct answer is (A). Using proportionalities to convert the total weight after summing, we have 132 lb + 11 lb + 44 lb = 187 lbs. So, then

$$\frac{1 \text{ kg}}{2.2 \text{ lb}} = \frac{x \text{ kg}}{187 \text{ lb}}$$

$$\frac{1 \text{ kg} \times 187 \text{ lb}}{2.2 \text{ lb}} = x \text{ kg}$$

$$x \text{ kg} = 85 \text{ kg}$$

84. The correct answer is (B). Simply convert to a common denominator and add (see Answer 19):

$$\left(\frac{3}{4}\right)^2 = \frac{3^2}{4^2} = \frac{9}{16}$$

$$3^2 = 9$$

$$\sqrt{\frac{49}{256}} = \frac{\sqrt{49}}{\sqrt{256}} = \frac{\sqrt{7 \times 7}}{\sqrt{2 \times 2 \times 2 \times 2 \times 2 \times 2 \times 2 \times 2}}$$

$$= \frac{7}{\sqrt{2^8}} = \frac{7}{2^4} = \frac{7}{16}$$

Therefore,

$$\left(\frac{3}{4}\right)^2 + 3^2 + \sqrt{\frac{49}{256}} = x$$

$$\frac{9}{16} + \frac{9 \times 16}{16} + \frac{7}{16} = x$$

$$x = \frac{160}{16} = 10$$

85. The correct answer is (C). The equation of a line is $y = mx + b$ (see Answers 26–28), where m is the slope and b is the y-intercept. Therefore:

$$y = mx + b$$
$$y = -2x + \sqrt{2}$$

86. The correct answer is (D). Simplify the numerator; then, divide the result by the denominator:

$$250,000 \times 0.018 = 4,500.000. = 4,500$$
$$\frac{4,500}{0.15} = 30,000.00$$
$$= 30,000$$

87. The correct answer is (A). If we use the law of exponents, $x^{-3} = \frac{1}{x^3}$, then:

$$\frac{1}{x^3} = \frac{1}{27}$$
$$x^3 = 27$$
$$x = \sqrt[3]{27} = \sqrt[3]{3 \times 3 \times 3}$$
$$= 3$$

88. The correct answer is (A). Corresponding sides of similar triangles are related by the same ratio. Therefore,

$$\frac{J}{K} = \text{ratio of one side}$$

$$\frac{H}{I} = \text{ratio of second side}$$

$$\frac{J}{K} = \frac{H}{I}$$

$$I = \frac{KH}{J}$$

89. The correct answer is (A). If drug A is 20% of the compound, then drug A is 20% of 500 g.

$$\frac{20\%}{100\%} \times 500 = \text{grams of drug A}$$

$$\frac{10,000}{100} = \text{grams of drug A} = 100$$

90. The correct answer is (B). Drugs A and B represent 20% and 5%, respectively, of the compound. Therefore, 25% of 500 g is the amount of drugs A and B.

$$\frac{20}{100}+\frac{5}{100}\times 500\,\text{g}=\text{grams of drugs A and B}$$

$$\frac{12,500}{100}=\text{grams of drugs A and B}=125\,\text{g}$$

91. The correct answer is (D). Drugs B and C represent 5% and 75% of the compound. Therefore, 80% of 500 g is the amount of drugs B and C.

$$\frac{5}{100}+\frac{75}{100}\times 500\,\text{g}=\text{grams of drugs B and C}$$

$$\frac{40,000}{100}=\text{grams of drugs B and C}=400$$

92. The correct answer is (A). Drugs A, B, and C represent 20%, 5%, and 75% of the compound, which, when summed, make up 100% of the compound. Therefore, 100 g of drugs A, B, and C are in 100 g of the compound.

93. The correct answer is (B). The ratios A:B:C are 20%:5%:75%. If 5 is the lowest common denominator, then:

$$\frac{20}{5}:\frac{5}{5}:\frac{75}{5} \text{ or, 4:1:15}$$

94. The correct answer is (D). If this problem is approached as a proportion, then the product of the means divided by one of the extremes equals the other extreme. Initially, isolate the extreme g_bM_b:

$$\frac{B-p}{q}=\frac{g_aM_b}{g_bM_a}$$

$$g_bM_a=\frac{(g_aM_b)(q)}{B-p}$$

Again, treat the equation as a proportion and isolate the extreme (g_b):

$$g_b=\frac{(g_aM_b)(q)}{(B-p)(M_a)}$$

that on rearrangement, yields

$$g_b=\left[\frac{q}{B-p}\right]\left[\frac{M_b(g_a)}{M_a}\right]$$

95. The correct answer is (D). From the equation for a straight line (see Answers 26–28), $y=mx+b$:

	y-intercept (b)	slope (m)	x-intercept (y = 0)
Equation 1	4	+3	$-\frac{4}{3}$
Equation 2	−4	+3	$\frac{4}{3}$

96. The correct answer is (A). To solve simultaneous equations, express the first equation in terms of a single unknown term (I). Then, substitute this value into the second equation and solve for the second unknown (II). After solving for the second unknown, substitute its value back into the first equation and solve for the remaining unknown term (III):

(I) $30=a+3b-70$

$a=30-3b+70$

(II) $3a+5b=100$

$3(30-3b+70)+5b=100$

$90-9b+210+5b=100$

$-4b=100-210-90$

$4b=200$

$b=50$

(III) $30=a+3b-70$

$30=a+3(50)-70$

$30=a+150-70$

$a=-50$

97. The correct answer is (B). The question is really asking what is the total volume used. This is the total volume of a dose times the number of doses, which is then expressed in milliliters:

$$\frac{2 \text{ tablespoonfuls}}{\text{dose}} \times \frac{2 \text{ doses}}{\text{day}} \times 10 \text{ days} = \text{total volume}$$

$$40 \text{ tablespoonfuls} \times \frac{15 \text{ ml}}{\text{tablespoonful}} = 600 \text{ ml}$$

98. The correct answer is (D). This problem is solved with proportions; however, because we will be dividing the total weight into smaller units, the weight should be converted to a smaller unit to minimize the number of decimal places of which we will have to keep track:

$$0.060 \text{ g} \times \frac{1{,}000 \text{ mg}}{1 \text{ g}} = 60 \text{ mg}$$

$$\frac{60 \text{ mg}}{125 \text{ tablets}} = \frac{x \text{ mg}}{\text{tablet}}$$

$$0.480 \text{ mg} = \frac{x \text{ mg}}{\text{tablet}}$$

99. The correct answer is (C). This is a conversion problem, which again, is easiest to solve by the use of proportions:

$$\frac{1 \text{ in.}}{2.54 \text{ cm}} = \frac{x \text{ in.}}{12.70 \text{ cm}}$$

$$\frac{12.70 \text{ cm} \times 1 \text{ in.}}{2.54 \text{ cm}} = x \text{ in.}$$

$$5 \text{ in.} = x$$

100. The correct answer is (A). To divide fractions, invert the second term and multiply:

$$\frac{1}{120} \div \frac{1}{150} = \frac{1}{120} \times \frac{150}{1} = \frac{150}{120}$$

Then, simplify and complete the multiplication:

$$\frac{150}{120} = \frac{15}{12} = \frac{5 \times 3}{4 \times 3} = \frac{5}{4}$$

$$\frac{5}{4} \times 50 = \frac{250}{4} = 62\frac{1}{2}$$

Chemistry

1.	D	21.	C	41.	C	61.	D	81.	D
2.	B	22.	B	42.	D	62.	A	82.	C
3.	B	23.	D	43.	B	63.	B	83.	B
4.	A	24.	D	44.	C	64.	C	84.	A
5.	B	25.	A	45.	C	65.	D	85.	B
6.	B	26.	A	46.	A	66.	A	86.	C
7.	B	27.	A	47.	D	67.	B	87.	D
8.	A	28.	B	48.	A	68.	C	88.	D
9.	C	29.	D	49.	D	69.	D	89.	A
10.	B	30.	C	50.	A	70.	D	90.	C
11.	B	31.	C	51.	A	71.	C	91.	B
12.	C	32.	D	52.	C	72.	B	92.	D
13.	C	33.	B	53.	B	73.	A	93.	C
14.	C	34.	A	54.	A	74.	C	94.	C
15.	D	35.	C	55.	A	75.	A	95.	A
16.	D	36.	C	56.	A	76.	B	96.	B
17.	A	37.	C	57.	B	77.	D	97.	C
18.	D	38.	D	58.	B	78.	D	98.	D
19.	A	39.	A	59.	B	79.	C	99.	B
20.	D	40.	D	60.	B	80.	B	100.	A

1. **The correct answer is (D).** Alkanes are saturated hydrocarbons containing only carbon and hydrogen. They are usually straight-chained compounds and the carbon atom utilizes four sp^3 hybrid orbitals, forming a tetrahedral arrangement. Each bond angle is 109.5°, and the general formula is C_nH_{2n+2}; for example, when there is one C atom, then there are four H atoms, as in methane. Alkenes have the general formula C_nH_{2n}.

2. **The correct answer is (B).** With regard to phenol, electron-releasing substituents (e.g.,–CH_3) will decrease its acidity and lower the K_a. An electron-attracting substituent (e.g., –NO_2) will withdraw the ring electrons, relatively, and increase the acidity of phenol, resulting in a higher K_a. Thus, a nitro substituent in the ortho position will increase the K_a, whereas a methyl substituent in the same position would lower the K_a. Furthermore, the –OH substituent is strongly ortho and para directing.

3. **The correct answer is (B).** Using the pH concept, we have pH = $-\log[H^+]$ = $\log\left[\frac{1}{[H^+]}\right]$.

Furthermore, pOH = $\log\left[\frac{1}{[OH^-]}\right]$, and [H+][OH–] equals 10–14.

From these relations, pH + pOH = 14.

4. **The correct answer is (A).** Hematite (Fe_2O_3) has a molecular weight of 160. The percentage of elemental iron in hematite is given as follows:

$$\frac{2Fe}{Fe_2O_3} = \frac{2(56)}{160} \times 100\%$$
$$= 70\%$$

Note that there are two atoms of iron in Fe_2O_3.

5. **The correct answer is (B).**

$$3H_2 \quad + \quad N_2 \quad \rightarrow \quad 2NH_3$$
(3 liters)   (1 liter)   (2 liters)

Setting up a direct proportion, that is,

$$\frac{2 \text{ liters of } NH_3}{2 \text{ liters of } H_2} = \frac{20 \text{ liters of } NH_3}{x \text{ liters of } H_2}$$

and solving for x will give an answer of 30 liters.

6. **The correct answer is (B).** The volume occupied by the gram-molecular weight of a gas under standard temperature and pressure conditions (i.e., 0°C and 760 mmHg) is called the gram-molecular volume. Hence, 1 mole of any gas under these conditions will occupy a volume of 22.4 liters. Be aware that 1 mole of the same gas may occupy a different volume at some other combination of temperature and pressure.

7. **The correct answer is (B).** The molecular weight of CO_2 is 44 g (i.e., $12 + 32$). Thus, the gram-molecular weight of CO_2 is 44 g, which occupies 22.4 liters at standard temperature and pressure. Therefore, the weight of 1 liter of CO_2 equals $\frac{(44 \text{ g})}{(22.4 \text{ liters})} = 1.9$ g. Since there are 2 liters of CO_2, the weight is 4 g.

8. **The correct answer is (A).** In acetylene, carbon forms two sp hybrid orbitals and thus enables itself to bind to two hydrogen atoms in a sigma bond. The carbon-carbon triple bond, however, is made up of one sigma bond and two pi bonds.

9. **The correct answer is (C).** The carbon in methane (CH_4) and the oxygen in water (H_2O) both form sp^3 hybrid orbitals. For carbon, the sp^3 hybridization results in four hybrid orbitals in which the axes are directed toward the corners of a tetrahedron. In the formation of water, oxygen bonds with two hydrogen atoms via its two unpaired electrons. The water molecule still has a tetrahedral shape; two corners are occupied by hydrogen atoms and the rest is occupied by the unshared pairs of electrons.

10. **The correct answer is (B).** In chemistry, the structural formula (e.g., $C_6H_{12}O_6$) reveals the numbers and types of atoms present in a molecule. In general, if not always, the arrangement of the different atoms can also be deduced from an examination of the structural formula. However, the structural formula of a molecule bears no relationship to the gram-molecular volume occupied by the gram-molecular weight of a gas under standard conditions.

11. **The correct answer is (B).** A knowledge of the chemical and physical properties of organic and inorganic compounds is important in understanding their chemical behavior. Organic compounds do exist as isomers and decompose upon heating at lower temperatures. They are also soluble in other organic solvents; that is, like dissolves like. However, organic compounds do not react with each other faster than inorganic compounds would.

12. **The correct answer is (C).** In radioactive disintegration, the emission of a beta particle does not change the atomic weight of the nucleus emitting the beta particle. This is due to the fact that the weight of a beta particle is extremely small. However, the atomic number increases by 1 and is thought to be the result of the breakdown of a neutron to a proton and an electron (beta particle). An alpha par-

ticle is a helium nucleus, and its emission, in contrast to that of a beta particle, results in a decrease of 4 units of atomic weight and 2 units of atomic number.

13. **The correct answer is (C).** The artificial conversion of one element into another (e.g., nitrogen into oxygen) is termed transmutation. Radioactive decay can occur spontaneously, resulting in the disintegration of the parent nucleus, with the consequent production of one or more daughter nuclei. This process is usually accompanied by the emanation (i.e., emission) of gamma rays. *Transformation* is a nonspecific term for changes in physical form.

14. **The correct answer is (C).** Gamma rays are high-energy X rays of very short wavelength that travel with the speed of light. Compared to alpha and beta rays, gamma rays are the most penetrating of the radiations emitted by radioactive compounds. Since they have no electrical charge, magnetic or electrical fields do not affect their path.

15. **The correct answer is (D).** Atomic fusion is the process of combining atoms to form elements of higher atomic weight. Frequently, tremendous energy is released during this process. Atomic fission is the process of splitting an atomic nucleus, which also results in the release of large amounts of energy. The process of electron capture results from the conversion of an orbital electron to a neutron, and the energy therein is negligible compared to that of atomic fusion and fission.

16. **The correct answer is (D).** Alcohols have the general formula ROH. While methanol and ethanol are the simplest and most easily recognized alcohols, glycerine is also an alcohol, even though it has three hydroxyl groups. Glycerine (or glycerol) is thus a polyalcohol and is widely used in pharmaceutical manufac-

turing. Sodium hydroxide (NaOH) is a base and not an alcohol. Remember that alcohols are organic compounds in which the hydroxyl group has been substituted for one or more hydrogen atoms in a hydrocarbon.

17. **The correct answer is (A).** Hydrogen chloride gas has a pungent smell, is extremely soluble in water, and reacts with ammonia to form white fumes of ammonium chloride. It is a colorless gas, but is not lighter than air. The density of the gas is greater than 1 g/cm^3 and is about 25% heavier than air.

18. **The correct answer is (D).** The halogen elements are fluorine, chlorine, bromine, iodine, and astatine. They comprise group VIIA of the periodic table. Note that these elements end in the suffix *-ine*; however, this does not mean that turpentine or nicotine belong to the halogen family.

19. **The correct answer is (A).** It can be stated that 1 Eq of any chemical is that quantity that is equivalent to 1 mole of replaceable hydrogen ions in an acid-base reaction. Thus, 1 mole of HCl contains 1 mole of replaceable hydrogen, and thus HCl has 1 Eq/mole. $HC_2H_3O_2$ is the formula for acetic acid, CH_3COOH. Clearly, only one hydrogen ionizes, and therefore acetic acid has 1 Eq/mole.

20. **The correct answer is (D).** Avogadro's law determines the relation between the properties of gases. In essence, it states that equal volumes of different gases at the same temperature and pressure contain the same number of molecules. Hence, if one keeps the temperature and pressure constant, the volume of any gas is proportional to its mass, and therefore to the number of gas molecules. Note that Charles's law states that the volume of a gas is directly proportional to the absolute temperature, provided that pressure remains constant. Boyle's law relates

the pressure and volume of a gas at constant temperature.

21. **The correct answer is (C).** There is one chiral center, and thus 2 possible isomers or 2 configurations.

22. **The correct answer is (B).** R from the Latin *rectus*, meaning right and S from the Latin *sinister*, meaning left.

23. **The correct answer is (D).** If one assumes complete ionization, 58.5 mg of sodium chloride will supply 23 mg of sodium ions. Similarly, to give 100 mg of sodium ions, it is required to supply $\frac{(100 \times 58.5)}{23}$ = 254 mg of sodium chloride crystals.

24. **The correct answer is (D).** One mEq of sodium chloride is equal to its gram-equivalent weight divided by 1,000. Hence, 1 mEq of sodium chloride equals 58.5 mg of sodium chloride and 2 mEq equals 117 mg. The concentration of this solution is 117 mg/ml.

25. **The correct answer is (A).** The milli equivalent is used primarily by the health profession to express the concentration of electrolytes in solution. Since Mr. Smith weighs 60 kg, he should receive 2×60 mEq of sodium chloride. One mEq of sodium chloride equals 58.5 mg of salt. Therefore, Mr. Smith requires $2 \times 60 \times 58.5$ mg of sodium chloride. The answer is 7,020 mg, or 7 g.

26. **The correct answer is (A).** Percent (%) means parts per hundred on a weight basis. Hence, a 0.9% solution translates to 0.9 g of sodium chloride per 100 ml of solution. Mr. Smith requires 7 g, which is $\frac{(7 \times 100 \text{ ml})}{0.9}$ of solution. This comes out to 777 ml of a 0.9% solution of sodium chloride.

27. **The correct answer is (A).** The pharmacist must be well versed with the different units used to express the strength or concentration of a particular drug in solution. This problem relates to a solution of sodium chloride that is half the

strength ordered. Hence, twice the volume must be supplied to give the same amount of sodium chloride ordered, that is, 777 ml $\times$ 2 = 1.5 liters.

28. **The correct answer is (B).** Osmotic pressure is directly affected by the total number of particles in solution. If one assumes complete dissociation, 1 mole of sodium chloride is composed of 2 mOsm of total particles (i.e., Na^+ and Cl^-).

29. **The correct answer is (D).** Osmotic activity is a function of the total number of particles present in a given solution, be they electrolytes or nonelectrolytes. Electrolytes, in general, will dissociate into their component ions, and hence the number of particles in solution will increase.

30. **The correct answer is (C).** This question illustrates the need to convert different units to arrive at the answer. One millimole of sodium chloride is equal to 2 mOsm of the salt. One millimole of sodium chloride is 58.5 mg. Since a 0.9% solution has 0.9 g (or 900 mg) of sodium chloride per 100 ml of solution, 900 mg of this sodium chloride is equal to $\frac{900}{58.5}$ or 15.4 mmole of sodium chloride. Now, since 1 mmole of sodium chloride is equal to 2 mOsm, 15.4 mmole equals 15.4 $\times$ 2 mOsm of sodium chloride. The answer is 31 mOsm.

31. **The correct answer is (C).** Hydrogen has an atomic number and an atomic weight of 1. Hence, it has one proton and one electron, which reside in the nucleus and K shell, respectively. Hydrogen does not have a neutron. The hydrogen isotopes deuterium and tritium have one and two neutrons in the nucleus, respectively.

32. **The correct answer is (D).** This problem relates to the concept of atomic weight and atomic number. The total number of protons equals the number of electrons in the shells. Beryllium has four electrons, and therefore four protons. The

total number of protons equals the atomic number, and therefore beryllium has an atomic number of 4. The total number of protons and neutrons comprises the atomic weight of the element. Beryllium has an atomic weight of 9, since it has five neutrons and four protons.

33. The correct answer is (B). Mercury forms bivalent mercuric (Hg^{2+}) and bivalent mercurous (Hg_2^{2+}) compounds, even though mercury has a valence of 2 and 1, respectively. Mercurous oxide is Hg_2O. Hg_2O_3, Hg_3O_2, and HgO_2 compounds are unknown.

34. The correct answer is (A). HNO_2 is nitrous acid. Nitronous acid, nitrate acid, and nitrite acid do not exist.

35. The correct answer is (C). The reverse of synthesis is decomposition, that is, the breakdown of a compound AB to yield an element A and an element B.

36. The correct answer is (C). When a particle is oxidized, it loses electrons. Therefore, oxidation is associated with electron loss. Conversely, reduction is associated with electron gain. Since oxidation and reduction processes occur simultaneously, loss and/or gain of electrons is to be expected. An oxidized particle therefore loses its (valence) electrons, which results in an increase in valence number.

37. The correct answer is (C). This is an exercise in the law of conservation of matter. Examination of the equation will show that the number of molecules of the reactants must equal the number of molecules of the products, that is,

$$2ABC_3 \qquad 2AB + 3C_2$$

Reactant	=	Product
2A		2A
2B		2B
6C		6C

38. The correct answer is (D). The oxygen molecule is diatomic (O_2). Ozone is a triatomic molecule (O_3) of oxygen; its properties are different from those of oxygen.

39. The correct answer is (A). It is common knowledge that oxygen gas is combustible; however, it cannot be overemphasized that oxygen *supports* combustion and does not burn by itself. Its lack of odor and color does not help in its quick identification.

40. The correct answer is (D). Hydrogen peroxide is H_2O_2. The word *peroxide* means that it contains one more oxygen atom than would normally be expected. Water (H_2O) is the simplest molecule formed between the atoms of oxygen and hydrogen. Two molecules of hydrogen peroxide decompose via the following reaction, yielding two molecules of water and one molecule of oxygen: $2H_2O_2 \rightarrow H_2O + O_2$.

41. The correct answer is (C). This problem deals with the concept of density. Since the gram is defined as the mass of 1 cm^3 (approximately 1 ml) of water at $4°C$, water has a density of 1 g/ml; 5,000 ml of water weigh 5,000 g.

42. The correct answer is (D). The student is expected to be familiar with the different units used in expressing the quantity of a given solute in a quantity of solvent or total solution. Molarity (M) is defined as the number of moles of solute per liter of solution. In contrast, molality is the number of moles of solute in 1 kg of solvent. You should also be aware that normality (N) is defined as the number of equivalents of solute per liter of solution.

43. The correct answer is (B). The molecular weight of NaOH is 40. Hence, 40 g of NaOH are equivalent to 1 mole of NaOH. Molarity is defined as the number of moles of solute per liter of solution. Therefore, 1 mole of NaOH dissolved in 1 liter of solution is a 1 M solution. Dissolving 1 mole in 400 ml would give a higher molarity, that is, an increase by a factor of 2.5.

44. **The correct answer is (C).** If you are still unclear about moles and molarity by the time you get to this question, a review is required. One mole of sodium hydroxide equals 40 g dissolved in 1 liter of solution. A 5 M (molar) solution would mean 5 × 40 g of sodium hydroxide dissolved in 1 liter of solution. Hence, 125 ml of this solution would contain (125 × 5 × 40) /1,000 of sodium hydroxide. The number of moles would now be easy to calculate: Just divide (125×5×40) g/1,000 by 40 g/mole. The answer is 0.625 mole.

45. **The correct answer is (C).** Since 125 ml of a 5 M solution contains 0.625 mole of sodium hydroxide, then 0.625 mole × 40 g/mole of sodium hydroxide yields 25 g of this base.

46. **The correct answer is (A).** A liter of pure water weighs 1 kg, if one assumes that water has a density of 1 g/ml. The molecular weight of water is 18 g/mole. One liter of pure water, therefore, contains $\frac{1,000 \text{ g}}{18 \text{ g/mole}}$ or 55.5 moles; 55.5 moles of water in a solution represents a molarity of 55.5.

47. **The correct answer is (D).** Colligative properties of solutions depend on the amount and concentration of the solute(s) in the solution. Hence boiling point, vapor pressure, and freezing point are all colligative properties. Specific gravity, which compares the weights of substances to that of water, is not a colligative property.

48. **The correct answer is (A).** Acid and base strengths are frequently expressed by pH values. The pH value of any number is defined as the negative logarithm (base 10) of that number; that is, if $x = 10^n$, then $\log x = n$ and the pH of x is $-n$. Since

pH $= -\log[H^+] = -\log[l]$, pH $= 0$. Note that a pH of 0 is not neutral. A pH of 7 represents neutrality.

49. **The correct answer is (D).** Since pOH + pH = 14 and pH = O, pOH equals 14. This would represent a very basic (strongly alkaline) solution.

50. **The correct answer is (A).** As indicated before, the pH value gives some idea of the strength of an acid or base. The higher the pH value, the lower the hydrogen ion concentration. A higher pH means that the substance is less acidic and more basic.

51. **The correct answer is (A).** Methane (CH_4) is the simplest saturated hydrocarbon of the alkane series. It is explosive when mixed with air, is the active component of natural gas, and is otherwise called marsh gas. Owing to its saturated character, methane is not important in addition reactions, but it will undergo substitution reactions.

52. **The correct answer is (C).** Esters have the general formula RCOOR. Ethyl acetate is $C_2H_5COOCH_3$. Nitroglycerine and methyl salicylate are both esters. Sodium formate (NaCOOH) is the salt of an organic acid and is therefore not an ester.

53. **The correct answer is (B).** Glucose is a monosaccharide. Dextran and cellulose are polysaccharides. Glyceryl stearate is a fatty acid and is widely employed in making soaps, for example, sodium stearate.

54. **The correct answer is (A).** Rayon, nylon, and Orlon are all synthetic fibers. Nylon is a synthetic protein, Orlon is a polyester fiber, and rayon is regenerated cellulose; however, cellulose is a nonsynthetic fiber.

55. **The correct answer is (A).** Werner Heisenberg showed that when one attempts to simultaneously determine the

position and momentum of an electron, an unavoidable uncertainty in both these parameters is created that cannot be resolved. Louis de Broglie advanced the hypothesis that electrons have wavelike characteristics, Planck is responsible for the foundations of quantum theory, and Bohr is known for his electronic theory of the atom.

56. **The correct answer is (A).** Four quantum numbers are necessary in order to fully characterize the electronic wave functions; these are n (the principle quantum number), l (the azimuthal quantum number), m (the magnetic quantum number), and s (the spin quantum number).

57. **The correct answer is (B).** Pauli's exclusion principle clearly demonstrates that an atom cannot exist in a state where two electrons in the same orbital have the same four quantum numbers. This principle is important when more and more electrons are added to the orbitals of the atoms in the periodic table.

58. **The correct answer is (B).** The student is expected to remember the atomic numbers of the first ten elements in the periodic table. Oxygen has eight electrons and its orbitals are filled according to a $1s^2 2s^2 2p^4$ electronic configuration. You should remember the minimum (or maximum) number of electrons that can occupy any orbital. These s, p, d, and f orbitals can be completely filled by 2, 6, 10, and 14 electrons, respectively.

59. **The correct answer is (B).** Carbon has 6 protons and, therefore, 6 electrons; however, its atomic weight is 12; that is, it has 6 protons and 6 neutrons. Hence, carbon has 6 protons, 6 electrons, and 6 neutrons. Remember that the atomic number is equal to the number of protons (or electrons) and that the atomic weight is the number of protons *and* neutrons in the nucleus.

60. **The correct answer is (B).** The $1s^2 2s^2 2p^2$ electronic distribution translates to 6 orbital electrons. Hence, this element has 6 electrons and therefore 6 protons. Carbon has 6 protons and 6 electrons. Beryllium has 4 electrons, helium has 2, and oxygen has 8. The element in question is carbon.

61. **The correct answer is (D).** Isotopes are atoms of elements having the same number of electrons, the same chemical characteristics, and the same valence. However, isotopes differ in their mass, that is, in the number of neutrons in the nucleus; for example, hydrogen (no neutrons) and tritium (two neutrons).

62. **The correct answer is (A).** Carbon-12 (ordinary carbon) has 6 electrons, 6 protons, and 6 neutrons. Carbon-14 is an isotope of carbon and differs only in mass (i.e., neutron number). Hence, carbon-14 has 2 extra neutrons when compared to natural carbon. In summary, carbon-12 has 6 electrons, 6 protons, and 6 neutrons; carbon-14 has 6 electrons, 6 protons, and 8 neutrons.

63. **The correct answer is (B).** Gamma-ray decay is associated primarily with the emission of electromagnetic radiation, that is, photons. The internal rearrangement of the atom is responsible for gamma-ray emission, and there are no changes in the nuclear mass (i.e., the number of protons and neutrons) of the atom. Alpha decay is associated with a decrease of 4 units of atomic weight.

64. **The correct answer is (C).** The angstrom (A°) is 1×10^{-10} m, or 1×10^{-8} cm, the average radius of an atom.

65. **The correct answer is (D).** The prefix *pyro-* indicates loss of water. In this example, a molecule of water is lost from two molecules of orthophosphoric acid to form pyrophosphoric acid. The prefixes *hypo-* and *per-* refer, respectively, to the

lowest and highest oxidation states. The prefix for the highest hydrated form is *ortho-*.

66. **The correct answer is (A).** Lead exists in the divalent (+2) and tetravalent (+4) oxidation states, where it is called the plumbus and plumbic ion, respectively. Copper also exists in two oxidation states, monovalent (+1) and divalent (+2).

67. **The correct answer is (B).** The alkaline-earth metals comprise group IIA of the periodic table. Phosphorus is not one of the elements in this group. Gypsum and plaster of paris are sulfate salts of calcium, the most abundant and useful element of group IIA. Plaster of paris is used to make plaster and surgical casts.

68. **The correct answer is (C).** Hydrogen sulfide gas not only smells obnoxious to the user, but it is also extremely toxic. It is a colorless gas, denser than air, and somewhat soluble in water; hence, the preparation and use of this gas should be carefully monitored.

69. **The correct answer is (D).** CH_3COOH follows the general formula RCOOH, which represents an organic acid. This particular organic acid is acetic acid, commonly called vinegar. Aqua fortis is the common name for nitric acid. Aqua regia is a mixture of nitric and hydrochloric acids, while muriatic acid is commercially produced hydrochloric acid.

70. **The correct answer is (D).** Baking soda is sodium bicarbonate, $NaHCO_3$. Sodium carbonate (Na_2CO_3) is washing soda and is used as a water softener. $Na_2B_4O_7$ is borax, while magnesium sulfate ($MgSO_4$) is known as Epsom salts.

71. **The correct answer is (C).** HOCl is hypochlorous acid, formed from the initial reaction of chlorine gas and water. Most bleaching agents (e.g., Clorox) act by the release of hypochlorous acid into

solution. Chloroform is an organic solvent ($CHCl_3$). Brine is the form of sodium chloride found in combination with sea water, while tincture of iodine is an alcoholic preparation containing iodine.

72. **The correct answer is (B).** Alkenes have double bonds. This double bond is made up of one pi bond and one sigma bond. In organic chemistry there are no alpha bonds, but there are alpha-designated carbon atoms.

73. **The correct answer is (A).** $RCONH_2$ are amides, the simplest member being formamide ($HCONH_2$). Acid anhydrides have the general formula $(RCO)_2O$, amines are generally RNH_2, while azides have the general formula $RCON_3$.

74. **The correct answer is (C).** An enzyme usually has the suffix *-ase*, sugar usually ends in *-ose*, while a carboxyl group would end in *-ate*.

75. **The correct answer is (A).** A tertiary (3°) alcohol has all of its alcohol carbon hydrogens substituted for other organic substituents; a secondary (2°) alcohol has only one hydrogen attached to the alcohol carbon; and a primary (1°) alcohol has only two hydrogens attached to the alcohol carbon. CH_3OH is methanol, which has only hydrogen attached to the alcohol carbon.

76. **The correct answer is (B).** Vinyl usually refers to the $CH_2 = CH$ radical. Thus, methyl vinyl ketone is $CH_3COCH = CH_2$. Ethyl vinyl ketone is $CH_3CH_2COCH = CH_2$. Butyric acid is $CH_3CH_2CH_2COOH$, whereas $CH_3OCH_2CH = CH_2$ is methyl allyl ether.

77. **The correct answer is (D).** An organic acid is usually identified by the longest hydrocarbon chain, with the carboxyl carbon as carbon number 1. Changing the suffix from *-ane* to *-ol* would make it an alcohol and not an acid.

78. **The correct answer is (D).** $CH_3(CH_2)_8CH_3$ has ten carbon atoms; hence, it is called decane. Nonane has nine carbon atoms, while octane has only eight. Undecane is $C_{11}H_{24}$, and there are thus eleven carbon atoms in this saturated hydrocarbon.

79. **The correct answer is (C).** Atoms in double- or triple-bonded systems are rigid and not free to rotate around these bonds. Furthermore, ring systems have an aromatic character, and the atoms in these systems are also not free to rotate around their bonds. Only atoms connected by single bonds rotate around their sigma bonds.

80. **The correct answer is (B).** The carbonium ions, by definition, are atoms that contain a carbon atom with only six electrons. They are classified as primary, secondary, and tertiary ions, as in the classification of the organic alcohols. Since the stability of a carbonium ion is greatly increased by charge dispersal, a tertiary carbonium ion, which has three alkyl groups, is more stable than a secondary carbonium ion, which has two alkyl groups. The more stable the carbonium ion, the more easily it is formed.

81. **The correct answer is (D).** Benzene is a planar molecule; that is, all its atoms lie in the same plane. There are pi electron clouds above and below the plane of the ring, making it a rigid molecule with the formula C_6H_6. Each carbon atom lies at an angle of a regular six-sided figure, or hexagon. The bond angle is therefore 120°.

82. **The correct answer is (C).** Aldehyde and ketones have the carbonyl (—C = 0) functional group. The carbonyl carbon is joined to three other atoms by sigma bonds; there is also an overlap of a pi bond. The carbon hybridization orbitals are sp^2, and the molecule is planar, with bond angles of 120°.

83. **The correct answer is (B).** With regard to chemical reactivity and nucleophilic displacement, nucleophilic substitution occurs more readily at an acyl carbon (i.e., —RCO) than at a saturated carbon. Hence, a compound having a carbonyl group would be more prone to undergo nucleophilic substitution; for example, amides would be more prone than amines, acid chlorides more than alkyl chlorides, and esters more than ethers.

84. **The correct answer is (A).** Glycols are polyalcohols, usually containing two hydroxyl groups. These are saturated compounds, the simplest being ethylene glycol, CH_2OHCH_2OH. The suffix *-ol* should remind you that we are dealing with alcohols.

85. **The correct answer is (B).** The Grignard reagent is unique owing to its high reactivity. Its general formula is RMgX, and it is formed by reacting an alkyl halide with metallic magnesium in ether. The carbon-magnesium bond is highly polar but distinctly covalent (i.e., sharing of electrons); however, the magnesium-halogen bond is ionic in character.

86. **The correct answer is (C).** Organic molecules are such that reactants must be optically active in order for the products to be optically active. The converse, that is, the relation between inactive reactants and inactive products, is also correct. However, the products of optically active reactants may not show such activity, and this is due to racemic modification of the isomers.

87. **The correct answer is (D).** CH_4 is methane, and $-CH_3$ is the methyl radical of this alkane. CH_2 or methylene exists as a discrete molecule and is highly reactive. Methanol is formaldehyde, the former being the International Union of Pure and Applied Chemistry (IUPAC) nomenclature and the latter being the common name. Mesyl is the shortened

form of the methyl sulfonyl radical and deals with sulfonic acid chemistry.

88. **The correct answer is (D).** The Diels-Alder reaction is important because the end product of the reactants, a diene and a dienophile, is a six-membered ring. The diene usually possesses electron-releasing groups, while the dienophile (an αβ-unsaturated carbonyl compound) is associated with electron-withdrawing functional groups. Note that the Diels-Alder reaction is a reaction between a conjugated diene and an α-unsaturated carbonyl compound.

89. **The correct answer is (A).** Disaccharides, on hydrolysis, yield two monosaccharides. Sucrose (cane sugar) will yield glucose and fructose. Maltose (malt sugar) will yield two molecules of glucose, while lactose (milk sugar) will yield glucose and galactose. Amylose is a water-soluble fraction of starch, a polysaccharide.

90. **The correct answer is (C).** Amino acids have the general formula $RCHNH_2COOH$. The amino acid with the simplest structure is NH_2CH_2COOH, or glycine. Tyrosine is an aromatic amino acid, whereas arginine is a basic amino acid. Methionine is an amino acid containing an atom of sulfur.

91. **The correct answer is (B).** Aryl halides are compounds in which the halogens are attached directly to the aromatic ring, for example, bromobenzene (C_6H_5Br). Alkyl halides are not only the saturated form of the halogen-containing compounds, for they also compose the substituted alkyl group, for example, vinyl chloride.

92. **The correct answer is (D).** The catalytic addition of oxygen to ethylene $(CH_2 = CH_2)$ results in the formation of ethylene oxide, which has the structure:

$$CH_2 \underset{O}{\diagdown\diagup} CH_2$$

Ethylene oxide is therefore an epoxide, whereas ethylene is an alkene.

93. **The correct answer is (C).** Amines have the general formula RNH_2. Primary amines have the formula RNH_2, secondary amines have the formula R_2NH, and tertiary amines have the formula R_3N. RNH is an amine radical and lacks either an R group or a hydrogen atom.

94. **The correct answer is (C).** One hundred percent alcohol (or 200 proof alcohol) is absolute alcohol or water-free alcohol. Methanol is synonymous with wood alcohol. Absolute alcohol absorbs various amounts of water from the atmosphere and must be stored accordingly.

95. **The correct answer is (A).** The simplest member of the fused-ring hydrocarbon family is naphthalene, which has two benzene rings. Anthracene has three fused benzene rings, just like phenanthrene.

96. **The correct answer is (B).** CH_3OH is the formula for an organic alcohol commonly known as methanol. Menthone is a long-chained organic compound (i.e., a terpene) with a keto group, whereas mesitol is trimethyl phenol, an alkyl-substituted aryl alcohol. Menthol is a cyclic alcohol derived from mint oils.

97. **The correct answer is (C).** Tollen's reagent contains $[Ag(NH_3)_2]^+$, the silver ammonium ion. Oxidation of an aldehyde to an acid is accompanied by the formation of a silver mirror. The latter is the result of the reduction of the soluble silver ion to yield free silver metal.

98. **The correct answer is (D).** Ammonia has the formula NH_3. Nitrogen uses four sp^3 orbitals in forming this molecule; they are directed toward the corners of a regular tetrahedron, with one orbital containing a pair of electrons. The other three each contain a single electron.

99. **The correct answer is (B).** By converting an organic acid to an acid chloride, we can produce a substance from which we can form esters and amides. Acid chlorides are much more reactive than their original acid and are therefore quite useful. Because of their reactivity, thionyl chloride and the chlorides of phosphorus are commonly employed in the preparation of acid chlorides. Note that these compounds have sulfur or phosphorus as the inorganic element. Ethyl chloride is a substituted halogenated hydrocarbon and plays no role in the preparation of such acid chlorides.

100. **The correct answer is (A).** All monosaccharides are reducing sugars, that is, they reduce Tollen's or Fehling's reagent. These monosaccharides can be aldo or keto sugars. Glucose is a monosaccharide and hence a reducing sugar. Most disaccharides are reducing sugars as well. Even though sucrose is a disaccharide, it does not reduce Tollen's or Fehling's solution.

Verbal Ability

1.	B	15.	B	29.	D	43.	B	57.	A
2.	B	16.	A	30.	C	44.	B	58.	D
3.	C	17.	C	31.	A	45.	C	59.	C
4.	A	18.	C	32.	A	46.	A	60.	B
5.	D	19.	D	33.	A	47.	D	61.	D
6.	D	20.	B	34.	C	48.	B	62.	B
7.	A	21.	A	35.	B	49.	B	63.	D
8.	C	22.	C	36.	C	50.	D	64.	A
9.	A	23.	B	37.	B	51.	B	65.	C
10.	A	24.	A	38.	A	52.	A	66.	C
11.	D	25.	D	39.	D	53.	A	67.	C
12.	C	26.	D	40.	B	54.	D	68.	B
13.	B	27.	B	41.	A	55.	D	69.	D
14.	D	28.	B	42.	D	56.	B	70.	B

1. **The correct answer is (B).** SECONDARY (n.)—one occupying a subordinate or auxiliary position rather than that of a principal. *Subordinate* (n.)—one that is placed in or occupying a lower class, rank, or position.

2. **The correct answer is (B).** ASLEEP (adj., adv.)—into a state of inactivity, sluggishness, or indifference. *Defunct* (adj.)—no longer living, existing, or functioning.

3. **The correct answer is (C).** COARSE (adj.)—of ordinary or inferior quality or value. *Crude* (adj.)—rough or inexpert in plan or execution.

4. **The correct answer is (A).** AMATEUR (n.)—one who engages in a pursuit, study, science, or sport as a pastime rather than as a profession. *Dabbler* (n.)—one who dabbles—as (adj.): one not deeply engaged in or concerned with something.

5. **The correct answer is (D).** UNDERVALUE (v.)—to value, rate, or estimate below the real worth. *Depreciate* (v.)—to lower in estimation or esteem.

6. **The correct answer is (D).** PRIMARY (n.)—something that stands first in rank, importance, or value. *Basis* (n.)—a supporting element; foundation.

7. **The correct answer is (A).** ANNOUNCEMENT (n.)—a public notification or declaration; a piece of formal stationery designed for a social or business announcement. *Mail* (n.)—materials, such as letters and packages, handled in a postal system.

8. **The correct answer is (C).** JAIL (n.)—a place of confinement for people held in lawful custody. *Lockup* (n.)—a jail.

9. **The correct answer is (A).** WRECK (n.)—the broken remains of something wrecked or otherwise ruined. *Crash* (n.)—to fall or collide noisily; smash.

10. **The correct answer is (A).** PLEASURE (n.)—a source of delight or joy. *Joy* (n.)—a condition or feeling of great pleasure.

11. **The correct answer is (D).** UNDOUBTED (adj.)—not doubted; genuine; undisputed. *Authentic* (adj.)—conforming to fact and therefore worthy of trust.

12. **The correct answer is (C).** SCHNOOK (n.)—a stupid or unimportant person. *Dunce* (n.)—one who is slow-witted or stupid.

13. **The correct answer is (B).** RETREAT (n.)—an act or a process of withdrawing, especially from what is difficult, dangerous, or disagreeable. *Charge* (v., n.)—to rush forward in or as in a violent attack.

14. **The correct answer is (D).** LINCOLN (n.)—Abraham Lincoln 1809–1865, sixteenth president of the United States (1861–65), known for his honesty and loyalty. *Genuine* (adj.)—free from hypocrisy or dishonesty.

15. **The correct answer is (B).** MOBILE (adj.)—capable of moving or being moved. *Running* (n., v.)—the act or action of one who runs.

16. **The correct answer is (A).** RADIO (n.)—the wireless transmission and reception of electric impulses or signals by means of electromagnetic waves. *Frequency* (n.)—the number of repetitions per unit time of a complete waveform.

17. **The correct answer is (C).** WIFE (n.)—a female partner in a marriage. *Son* (n.)—a male offspring.

18. **The correct answer is (C).** FEET (n.)—the terminal part of the vertebrate leg on which an individual stands. *Head* (n., adj., v.)—the upper most or forward most part of the body.

19. **The correct answer is (D).** ADDICT (v.)—to devote or surrender (oneself) to something habitually or obsessively. *Morphine* (n.)—an organic compound that is addictive; used for pain relief.

20. **The correct answer is (B).** BUTLER (n.)—the chief male servant of a household who has charge of other employees, receives guests, directs the serving of meals, and performs various personal services. *Valet* (n.)—to act as a personal servant.

21. **The correct answer is (A).** LANE (n.)—a relatively narrow way or track. *Roadway* (n.)—the strip of land over which a road passes.

22. **The correct answer is (C).** PIG (n.)—a young swine not yet sexually mature. *Porcine* (adj.)—relating to or suggesting swine.

23. **The correct answer is (B).** VICTORY (n.)—the overcoming of an enemy or antagonist. *Conquest* (n.)—the act or process of conquering.

24. **The correct answer is (A).** AGILE (adj.)—marked by ready ability to move with quick easy grace. *Supple* (adj.)—to make flexible or pliant.

25. **The correct answer is (D).** FERVOR (n.)—intensity of feeling or expression. Mute (n., adj.)—to tone down.

26. **The correct answer is (D).** DUNCE (n.)—a person dull or weak in intellect. *Brainy* (adj.)—having a well-developed intellect.

27. **The correct answer is (B).** ODD (adj.)—deviating from what is ordinary, usual, or expected. *Strange* (adj.)—not native to or naturally belonging to a place.

28. **The correct answer is (B).** OVOLO (n.)—a rounded convex molding. *Molding* (n.)—a decorative plane or curved strip used for ornamentation or finishing.

29. **The correct answer is (D).** EXPECT (v.)—to regard something as probable or likely. COUNT (v.)—to rely or depend on someone or something.

30. **The correct answer is (C).** DEPART (v.)—to go away; leave. *Withdraw* (v.)—to remove oneself from participation.

31. **The correct answer is (A).** BATMAN (n.)—comic book character name. *Comics* (n.)—the parts of a newspaper devoted to comic strips, a book of comic strips.

32. **The correct answer is (A).** PRODIGALITY (n.)—profuse generosity. *Parsimonious* (adj.)—frugal to the point of stinginess.

33. **The correct answer is (A).** PROGRESS (v.)—to advance or proceed. Headway (n.)—motion or rate of motion in a forward direction.

34. **The correct answer is (C).** PROGRAMMA (n.)—an edict published for public information. *Agenda* (n.)—a list, an outline, or a plan of things to be considered or done.

35. **The correct answer is (B).** STARVE (v.)—to suffer or die from extreme or prolonged lack of food. *Suckle* (v.)—to give milk to from the breast.

36. **The correct answer is (C).** INNING (n.)—a period of play in baseball during which each team has a turn at bat. *Frame* (n., v.)—something composed of parts fitted together and united.

37. **The correct answer is (B).** NOVEL (adj.)—strikingly new, unusual, or different. *Neoteric* (adj.)—recent in origin.

38. **The correct answer is (A).** SOFT (adj.)—smooth or fine to the touch. *Pulpy* (adj.)—the soft part of fruit.

39. **The correct answer is (D).** RUDE (adj.)—being in a crude, rough, unfinished condition. Crude (adj.)—marked by the primitive, gross, or elemental.

40. **The correct answer is (B).** LOVED (v.)—to have a deep feeling of affection and solicitude toward. *Adored* (v.)—to be extremely fond of.

41. **The correct answer is (A).** CONFIRM (v.)—to support or establish the certainty or validity of. *Contradict* (v.)—to resist or oppose in argument.

42. **The correct answer is (D).** TAUNT (v.)—to reproach in a mocking, insulting, or contemptuous manner. *Deride* (v.)—to laugh at contemptuously.

43. **The correct answer is (B).** MISER (n.)—one who lives very meagerly in order to hoard money. *Spendthrift* (n.)—one who spends improvidently or wastefully.

44. **The correct answer is (B).** MILKSOP (n.)—a timid man or boy considered childish or unassertive. *Doormat* (n.)—one who submits without protest to abuse or indignities.

45. **The correct answer is (C).** RAMPART (n.)—a fortification consisting of an embankment. *Bastion* (n.)—a projecting part of a fortification.

46. **The correct answer is (A).** IMPEND (v.)—to be imminent or about to happen. *Loom* (v.)—to take shape as an impending occurrence.

47. **The correct answer is (D).** PERSUADABLE (adj.)—being susceptible to persuasion. *Receptive* (adj.)—able or inclined to receive.

48. **The correct answer is (B).** EXTERNAL (adj.)—relating to, existing on, or connected with the outside or an outer part; exterior. *Internal* (adj.)—existing or situated within the limits or surface of something.

49. **The correct answer is (B).** GROVELING (adj.)—totally submissive. *Domineering* (adj.)—inclined to domineer.

50. **The correct answer is (D).** DOODLE (n.)—a trifler; a simple fellow. *Imbecile* (n.)—a mentally deficient person.

51. The correct answer is (B). For the first substitution, we need a choice that passes some judgment about the students who do not repay their loans. For the second element, we need a choice that will show a logical connection between the failure of some students to repay loans and the later availability of loan money for others.

52. The correct answer is (A). The "Although…" structure requires a contrast between the thoughts in the first clause and those in the second clause.

53. The correct answer is (A). There are two keys to this question. First, the "Contrary to…" structure sets up a contrast between peace-loving and something else. Additionally, you'll want a pair of words that will apply to both the warriors and the gods, bringing them into a parallel relationship. Choice (A) does this by first contrasting peace-loving astronomers with formidable warriors, then establishing a parallel between the formidable warriors and the vengeful gods.

54. The correct answer is (D). You can eliminate choices (B) and (C) on the basis of their second elements. And you can probably see that choice (D) is a good answer because it provides the needed contrast indicated by the introductory word "Despite" and supplies a second element that could be used to describe the feeling of the Academy.

55. The correct answer is (D). All but one of the choices can be eliminated on the basis of the first substitution. Notice that the question refers to the "delightful" characters of Irving. Only "charm" is consistent with such a judgment. Additionally, only "borrowed," of all the possible second elements, provides the logical contrast required by the second part of the sentence.

56. The correct answer is (B). The "Although" that introduces the sentence requires a contrast in the second portion of the sentence; only choice (B) provides this.

57. The correct answer is (A). The sentence starts with a thought-reverser, so we know that the correct choice will describe something unexpected given the amount of money invested. The second blank will be a logical continuation of the first blank as the verb "continues" indicates.

58. The correct answer is (D). This sentence starts with a thought-reverser, so we know that bats are going to be something that is the opposite of aggressive and rabid.

59. The correct answer is (C). In this sentence a thought-extender and a though-reverser are the logical keys. The first blank needs a word that continues the idea of "vagueness"; the second blank is unlike the first and must therefore be something close to an opposite.

60. The correct answer is (B). This sentence has a thought-reverser and thought-extender as its logical structure. The sentence says that the lawyer argues only what is central, eliminating something. Logically, what is eliminated is what is not central, so you should look for a word that is the opposite of central.

61. The correct answer is (D). This sentence contains a thought-reverser and a thought-extender. The thought-reverser is signaled by the phrase "even though." Since people persist, even though the government does something, the government must be trying to stop the belief in extraterrestrial life. The second blank requires a thought-extender, something that extends the idea of personal, and reverses the idea of godless.

62. The correct answer is (B). This sentence contains a thought-reverser and a thought-extender. The "in fact" in the second part of the sentence is the clue that tells you that the theory of the breakup of the continents is somehow changed. We are therefore looking for the opposite of occurring in stages or something close to it. The second blank requires an extension of that idea.

63. **The correct answer is (D).** This question contains a thought-extender and a thought-reverser as its logical elements. The first blank must parallel the idea that someone was the life of the party. His wife must be the opposite of the life of the party, or silent.

64. **The correct answer is (A).** This sentence begins with a thought-extender and then reverses the idea. The first blank needs an adjective related to "offhand" that could be applied to "remarks." This becomes a vocabulary question because you must know the meanings of all four of the first elements. All four answers make some sense, so it is a matter of substituting each pair to make sure that the logic of the sentence is maintained. If you know the meaning of "flippant," you don't have to look any further. He was flippant, but his attitude masked a serious nature.

65. **The correct answer is (C).** This question starts with a thought-reverser, "although." Choice (A) does not reverse the idea. The same is true of choice (D). Choices (B) and (C) remain possibilities, so test the second elements. The faculty might harbor her ideas, but they can't be doing it in defense of her seniority. Choice (C) works well. The faculty implements her ideas although they do not agree with her.

66. **The correct answer is (C).** This question contains a type of thought-reversal. Before looking at the choices, you already know you need a word that prevents time from being "idle."

67. **The correct answer is (C).** You cannot eliminate any of the choices on the grounds of usage, since each, when substituted into the sentence, will create phrases. The key to the sentence is the word "life." The field of study that completes the first blank must be a science that not only studies but directs the course of life, as indicated by the word "tamper."

68. **The correct answer is (B).** The logical key to this question is a double-reversal. "Although" sets up a contrast between the idea in the first clause and the idea in the second clause. But the second clause contains the word "little," which functions as a negative. So the blanks will actually extend the thought expressed in the first clause. The first blank is an extender of the concept of literature that instructs as well as entertains, so you should look for an adjective that describes this type of literature. All of the first choices might describe literature, so you need to know that "didactic" means instructive.

69. **The correct answer is (D).** This is basically a vocabulary question. You do, however, have one clue to the meaning of the sentence. The sentence tells you that Western physicians are learning a procedure. Logically, they are doing this because it is desirable, so you should look for the word that has a positive connotation.

70. **The correct answer is (B).** The second blank is an extension of the first idea. You can eliminate choice (A) because the idea of hearing a melody does not explain why a chord is superfluous. You can eliminate choice (C) because the idea of hearing applause doesn't explain why a chord might be melodious. And you can eliminate choice (D) because hearing harmony doesn't explain why a chord might be versatile.

Critical Thinking Essay

Have someone you respect—a professor or a professional writer—read your essay. Then ask him or her to grade it based on the following scoring criteria:

SCORE POINT 5—SUPERIOR

The writer is in command of the conventions of language; makes very few, if any, mistakes in sentence formation, usage, and mechanics. Some evidence is shown of advanced or innovative techniques.

SCORE POINT 4—EFFECTIVE

On the whole, the writer correctly applies the conventions of language, though there are some mistakes in sentence formation, usage, or mechanics. However, none of these errors are serious enough to interfere with the overall flow of the response or with its meaning.

SCORE POINT 3—ADEQUATE

The writer is fairly successful in applying the conventions of language. Several mistakes in sentence formation, usage, or mechanics are present. While the density of these errors may interfere with the overall flow of the response, they do not interfere with its meaning.

SCORE POINT 2—MARGINAL

The writer is marginally successful in applying the conventions of language. Patterns of mistakes in sentence formation, usage, and mechanics significantly detract from the presentation. At times the meaning of the response may be weakened.

SCORE POINT 1—WEAK

The writer's achievement in applying the conventions of language is limited. Frequent and serious mistakes in sentence formation, usage, and mechanics make the response difficult to understand.

PART III

PREPARING FOR YOUR PHARMACY CAREER

CHAPTER 3   Pharmacy Education

CHAPTER 4   Admission Process

CHAPTER 5   Postgraduate Education

CHAPTER 6   Making Pharmacy Your Career

Pharmacy Education

OVERVIEW

- Accreditation of pharmacy education
- Institutions and programs
- Pharmacy students
- Components of pharmacy education
- Degrees offered
- Pre-pharmacy requirements
- Professional pharmacy curriculum
- Frequently asked questions about pharmacy education
- Summing it up

ACCREDITATION OF PHARMACY EDUCATION

Pharmacy colleges are accredited by the American Council on Pharmaceutical Education (ACPE). The ACPE was established in 1932 and is the national accrediting agency in pharmacy recognized by the Secretary of Education, U.S. Department of Education, and the Council on Postsecondary Accreditation (COPA). The ACPE is also a member of the Council of Specialized Accrediting Agencies.

The ACPE is an autonomous agency whose membership is derived through the American Association of Colleges of Pharmacy (AACP), the American Pharmaceutical Association (APhA), and the National Association of Boards of Pharmacy (NABP), with three members appointed by each of the respective associations. In addition, there is one member appointed from the American Council on Education (ACE). Also, a panel of public representatives serves in an advisory capacity to the council and provides public contribution to its proceedings. The American Foundation for Pharmaceutical Education provides major financial support for the council's general activities. The AACP, APhA, and NABP also provide annual support to sustain the council's activities. Colleges pay an annual fee to the ACPE to maintain their accreditation status and also to pay for related expenses once accredited.

A list of accredited degree programs is published annually by the ACPE and is available on request. Contact the American Council on Pharmaceutical Education (ACPE), 20 North Clark Street, Suite 2500, Chicago, IL 60602; Phone: (312)

chapter 3

135

664-3575; Fax: (312) 664-4652; E-mail: acpe-accredit.org; Web site: www.acpe-accredit.org.

You must graduate from a college or school of pharmacy that is accredited by the American Council on Pharmaceutical Education to be eligible to take the North American Pharmacy Licensure Examination™ (NAPLEX)® given by the state board of pharmacy in your state. Each state gives the examination, with the exception of California, which conducts its own examination. Students should contact their state to determine how the board examination is given and to ask any other questions concerning state requirements.

For more information, contact the National Association of Boards of Pharmacy (NABP), 1600 Feehanville Drive, Mount Prospect, IL 60056; Phone: (847) 391-4406; Fax: (847) 391-4502; E-mail: custserv@napb.net; Web site: www.napb.net.

INSTITUTIONS AND PROGRAMS

As of fall 2004, ninety-three U.S. colleges and schools of pharmacy are accredited or in pre-candidate status.

Although each college of pharmacy curriculum has the same basic courses, the variation occurs in the course sequence, credit hours per courses, elective courses, total number of hours required for graduation, and pre-pharmacy requirements.

In July 1997, the American Council on Pharmaceutical Education (ACPE) adopted new accreditation standards and guidelines that resulted in accreditation only for colleges or schools that offer the Pharm.D. Today, all schools of pharmacy have implemented the Pharm.D. degree as the only entry-level degree.

PHARMACY STUDENTS

The AACP's annual Applicant Pool Survey indicated that from September 2003 through August 2004, ninety-three schools and colleges received 72,799 applications to first professional degree programs—an increase of 53.9 percent from the previous year. According to the survey, 62.0 percent of the applications were from women and 36.0 percent were from men. Applications from African Americans represented 8.4 percent of the total applications for 2004–05; applications from the Hispanic population, 3.7 percent; and applications from Native Americans, 0.5 percent. Of the applicants in 2004–05, 69.0 percent were submitted by students who had completed three or more years of postsecondary education; 29 percent had completed three or more years without earning a degree; 36.3 percent held a baccalaureate; 2.1 percent held a master's degree; and 0.5 percent held a doctorate.

The total number of professional degrees conferred in 2004 was 8,158. Women received 66.6 percent of the first professional degrees and men received 33.4 percent. Of the first professional degrees conferred, 4.8 percent earned B.S. degrees and 95.2 percent earned Pharm.D. degrees. Also, there were 986 post-B.S. Pharm.D. degrees awarded in 2004. The total number of M.S. degrees conferred was 651. There were 335 Ph.D. degrees awarded.

* Above data were compiled from the AACP Profile of Students Report, Fall 2004.

COMPONENTS OF PHARMACY EDUCATION

Pharmacy education can be divided into five distinct components:

1 Pre-pharmacy education, which requires two years at a minimum and may be taken at a junior college, community college, four-year college, or university. (Time may be reduced by taking an accelerated course load, although this is not necessarily recommended.)

2 Professional pharmacy education, which takes either three years (year-round Pharm.D. degree) or four years (Pharm.D. degree), must be taken at one of the ninety-three accredited schools or colleges of pharmacy in the United States to qualify to take the NAPLEX® examination for licensure.

3 Graduate education, which leads to an M.S. or Ph.D. degree.

4 Residency or fellowship programs after the Pharm.D. entry-level degree. These are one- or two-year professional experiences offered in several practice settings.

5 Professional continuing pharmaceutical education, which is a requirement for continued licensure as a pharmacist. Each state board of pharmacy has state-specific requirements. The majority of states require that pharmacists obtain 15 contact hours (1.5 C.E.U.) each year to maintain their licenses.

DEGREES OFFERED

The graduate degrees offered in the pharmaceutical sciences include the following:

1 Master of Science—M.S.

2 Doctor of Philosophy—Ph.D.

Many pharmacy colleges offer graduate programs at the master's and/or doctoral levels. The focus areas include the following:

- Medicinal chemistry
- Pharmaceutics
- Pharmacology
- Toxicology
- Pharmacokinetics

NOTE

There had been two professional pharmacy degrees offered by schools and colleges of pharmacy as the entry-level degree. However, schools now offer only the Pharm.D. as the entry-level degree.

- Drug metabolism
- Molecular modeling
- Nuclear pharmacy
- Health science administration
- Pharmacoeconomics
- Social and administrative pharmacy and health policy

There are several colleges of pharmacy that offer a joint Pharm.D./Ph.D. program. In these programs, students take all of their electives in the graduate school and must have either a previous B.S. degree in an area other than pharmacy or three years of pre-pharmacy with significant course work beyond the pre-pharmacy requirements to enter the program.

Another popular combined graduate program is the joint B.S./M.B.A. or Pharm.D./M.B.A. Students with the joint degree are attractive job candidates to the government, the pharmaceutical industry, and the chain-drug industry.

For information on graduate education programs and on joint undergraduate professional and graduate degree programs, contact the school or college of pharmacy that you are considering. You should also inquire about how many graduates enter residencies or fellowships after graduation.

PRE-PHARMACY REQUIREMENTS

Most pharmacy schools or colleges require two years of pre-pharmacy for entrance into the professional curriculum. Some programs have a 0–6 (pre-pharmacy/professional) program, whereas others have a 1–5, 2–4, or 3–4 program. A two-year pre-pharmacy curriculum includes either 60 semester hours or 90 quarter hours, depending on the particular program. The following two examples are for a program requiring two years of pre-pharmacy and one requiring three years of pre-pharmacy. The three-year pre-pharmacy requirements are for admission to the University of Tennessee College of Pharmacy and are provided for guidance only. Requirements for colleges of pharmacy vary; the major difference is in the number of required hours in physics, organic chemistry, and mathematics. Students should contact each institution for specific information about requirements.

Two Years of Pre-Pharmacy Requirements

TYPICAL PRE-PHARMACY CURRICULUM

Course	Semester Hours
General Chemistry	8
Organic Chemistry	8
General Biology/Zoology	8
Physics	4
Microbiology	4
English Composition	6
Communications/Speech (Interpersonal skills, not drama or theater)	3
Statistics	3
Fundamentals of Calculus	3
Social Science Electives (Psychology, Sociology, Economics, Anthropology, and Political Science)	6
Humanities Electives (Literature, Language, History, and Philosophy)	6
General Electives	7
TOTAL	66

Three Years of Pre-Pharmacy Requirements

PRE-PHARMACY CURRICULUM

UNIVERSITY OF TENNESSEE COLLEGE OF PHARMACY

The University of Tennessee's minimum requirements for admission to its College of Pharmacy are as follows:

1. Completion of 90 semester hours, with 66 semester hours of required pre-pharmacy courses and 26 semester hours of elective courses.

2. The PCAT is required at UT (see lists of colleges and schools for those that require the PCAT). A composite scaled score of 190 is required at UT; however, this score is not a competitive score.

3. A personal interview and three letters of reference are required.

4. A grade of C or above must be obtained in each required course.

Course	Semester Hours
General Chemistry	8
Organic Chemistry	8
General Biology/Zoology	8
Physics	4
Microbiology	4
English Composition	6
Communications/Speech (Interpersonal skills, not drama or theater)	3
Statistics	3
Fundamentals of Calculus	3
Social Science Electives (Psychology, Sociology, Economics, Anthropology, and Political Science)	6
Biochemistry	6
Immunology	3
Anatomy and Physiology	8
Humanities Electives (Literature, Language, History, and Philosophy)	6
General Electives	14
TOTAL	90

Note: One year of American History (high school or college level) is required for graduation from the University of Tennessee.

ALERT!

For information on pre-pharmacy requirements, graduate education programs, joint undergraduate professional, and graduate degree programs, contact the college or school of pharmacy you are considering.

PROFESSIONAL PHARMACY CURRICULUM

The pharmacy curriculum comprises basic science and clinical science courses. The following is an example of a Pharm.D. curriculum. This curriculum provides an example of the intensity and content of the pharmacy curriculum.

Doctor of Pharmacy Sample Curriculum

FIRST PROFESSIONAL YEAR

FALL SEMESTER

	Semester Hours	Lecture/Laboratory
ANAT 111 Anatomy	3	(2/2)
BIOC 111 Biochemistry	5	(4/2)
PHSC 112 Medicinal Chemistry I	3	(3/0)
PPE 132 Intro. Pharmacy & the Health-Care Environment	3	(2/2)
PHSC 111 Physical Pharmacy	3	(3/0)
PHSC 113 Pharmacy Math	1	(1/0)
Total Hours	18	(15/6)

SPRING SEMESTER

	Semester Hours	Lecture/Laboratory
PHSC 122 Medicinal Chemistry II	3	(3/0)
PHYS 121 Physiology	5	(4/1)
PHSC 123 Pharmaceutical Technology	5	(4/4)
MICR 211 Microbiology & Immunology	4	(3/2)
PPE 121 Basic Clinical & Communication Skills	2	(1/3)
Total Hours	19	(15/10)
FIRST YEAR TOTAL SEMESTER HOURS	37	

SECOND PROFESSIONAL YEAR

FALL SEMESTER

	Semester Hours	Lecture/Laboratory
PHAR 211 Pharmacology I	4	(3/2)
PHSC 212 Parenterals	2	(1/3)
PHSC 221 Biopharmaceutics	3	(3/0)
PPE 211 Professional Practice Management	2	(2/0)
PPE 224 Introductory Clerkship	1	(0/2)
Elective(s)	4	(varies)
Total Hours	16	(12/4)

SPRING SEMESTER

	Semester Hours	Lecture/Laboratory
PHAR 221 Pharmacology II	4	(4/0)
PPE 221 Self-care & Nonprescription Drugs	3	(3/0)
CLPH 311 Therapeutics I	4	(4/0)
PPE 222 Drug Information & Literature Evaluation	2	(1/2)
PHSC 233 Pharmacokinetics	3	(2/2)
CLPH 324/325 Community/ Institutional Rotation (May)	4	(0/10)
Elective(s)	2	(varies)
Total Hours	22	(14/14)
SECOND YEAR TOTAL SEMESTER HOURS	38	

THIRD PROFESSIONAL YEAR

FALL SEMESTER

	Semester Hours	Lecture/Laboratory
CLPH 312 Therapeutics II	4	(4/0)
CLPH 313 Therapeutics III	4	(4/0)
CLPH 314 Applied Therapeutics	2	(2/0)
CLPH 315 Applied Pharmacokinetics	3	(2/2)
PPE 213 Legal & Ethical Environment of Pharmacy	3	(3/0)
Elective(s)	2	(varies)
Total Hours	18	(16/2)

SPRING SEMESTER

	Semester Hours	Lecture/Laboratory
CLPH 321 Therapeutics IV	3	(3/0)
CLPH 322 Therapeutics V	3	(3/0)
PPE 223 Patient Assessment	2	(1/2)
CLPH 323 Applied Therapeutics II	2	(2/0)
PPE 324/325 Community/Institutional Rotation	4	(0/10)
Therapeutic Selective	2	(2/0)
Total Hours	16	(11/12)
THIRD YEAR TOTAL SEMESTER HOURS	34	

FOURTH PROFESSIONAL YEAR

FALL SEMESTER

	Semester Hours	Lecture/Laboratory
CLPH 411 Clinical Rotation I	4	(0/10)
CLPH 412 Clinical Rotation II	4	(0/10)
CLPH 413 Clinical Rotation III	4	(0/10)
CLPH 414 Clinical Rotation IV	4	(0/10)
CLPH 415 Clinical Rotation V	4	(0/10)
Total Hours	20	(0/50)

SPRING SEMESTER

	Semester Hours	Lecture/Laboratory
Rotation (selective)	4	(0/10)
Rotation (selective)	4	(0/10)
Rotation (selective)	4	(0/10)
Rotation (elective	4	(0/10)
Rotation (elective)	4	(0/10)
Total Hours	20	(0/50)
FOURTH YEAR TOTAL SEMESTER HOURS	40	

As you can see, there is a significant amount of basic science course work, including biochemistry, anatomy, physiology, and medical microbiology, as well as pharmaceutical chemistry and pharmacology, in the pharmacy curriculum. Other required courses may include nonprescription products, communication skills, toxicology, and drug literature evaluation.

The clinical science area of the curriculum deals with professional practice. The curriculum of the final professional year is oriented toward pharmacy practice. Students participate in rotations (professional experience program) where they apply what they have learned (basic and pharmaceutical sciences) to actual pharmacy practice. At rotation sites, students are educated by practicing pharmacists alongside medical, nursing, and other health-care students in a "health-care team approach."

Students can obtain rotation experience in such settings as community pharmacies, drug information centers, adult medical units, pediatric units, psychiatric units, ambulatory clinics, long-term care facilities, pharmaceutical manufacturing firms, and nuclear pharmacies. At these sites, students provide several services to patients, including dispensing medications, educating and monitoring patients about drug therapy, and conducting medication history interviews. Students may also serve as consultants, providing information to other health-care professionals about drug therapies.

Pharm.D. curricula require a minimum of 1,500 hours of professional practice experience. The University of Tennessee requires 1,960 hours of rotation experience. These hours are obtained by completing 12 one-month experiences of 160 hours per month.

ALERT!

For information on a pharmacy college's curriculum, write to the dean's office of the college in which you are interested. The addresses of accredited colleges of pharmacy in the United States are listed in the Appendix A.

FREQUENTLY ASKED QUESTIONS ABOUT PHARMACY EDUCATION

What are the job opportunities for a Doctor of Pharmacy graduate?

The Pharm.D. graduate is qualified for highly specialized fields.

Can the Pharm.D. candidate specialize in a chosen area?

Most Pharm.D. programs offer students the opportunity to take electives and develop emphasis in areas such as pharmacokinetics, metabolic support, nuclear pharmacy, pediatrics, drug information, mental health, geriatrics, infectious disease, home health care, community pharmacy, industrial pharmacy, and other specialties.

Are postdoctoral residencies available?

There are numerous residency options available to graduates, including general hospital pharmacy residencies, specialty residencies, clinical residencies, and fellowships. A general residency or clinical residency is normally completed before the fellowship. Residencies are currently accredited by the American Society of Health-System Pharmacists (ASHP), and several new residency programs are being developed in community and other ambulatory-care settings. Residency descriptions and information can be obtained from the ASHP. Details about residency programs in the community are available from the American Pharmaceutical Association.

How will future roles of pharmacists differ from present roles?

The financing and organization of health care is changing rapidly. As the health-care system changes, so do the professions within the system. New laws in several states permit pharmacists to become actively involved in the prescribing of medications (collaborative-care agreements). There will be a continuous evolution of the pharmacist's role from dispenser of medications to health practitioner—with greater control over the selection and administration of medicines. Managed care and the marketplace are dictating major changes in the health-care system, and pharmacy is responding to those needs.

Do the anticipated changes in roles for the future necessitate a change in education?

Education will meet the future needs of the pharmacy practitioner. Greater emphasis is being placed on high technology, wellness care, self-care, computer applications, and other innovations to prepare pharmacists for new responsibilities. Doctor of Pharmacy degree programs have evolved over the years in response to changing demands for specialized instruction and training. More pharmacists are continuing in postgraduate education after their Pharm.D. degree to prepare themselves for specialty areas of practice.

What factors should be considered when selecting a program for a professional pharmacy education?

Choosing a college or school of pharmacy is an extremely important and often difficult decision. Many factors should be evaluated, but the primary goal is to select the program that offers the highest quality of education and level of service. The institution's commitment to academic excellence and concern for students' needs are important selection criteria. The location and setting are also key factors.

SUMMING IT UP

- You must graduate from a college or school of pharmacy that is accredited by the American Council on Pharmaceutical Education to be eligible to take the NAPLEX®.

- Pharmacy education can be divided into five distinct components: pre-pharmacy education, professional pharmacy education, graduate education, residency or fellowship programs, and professional continuing pharmaceutical education.

- The Pharm.D. is the only entry-level degree offered by schools of pharmacy.

- Graduate degrees offered in the pharmaceutical sciences include the Master of Science (M.S.) and the Doctor of Pharmacy (Ph.D.).

Admission Process

OVERVIEW

- **Requirements for admission**
- **Health profession advisers**
- **Application process**
- **Pharmacy education costs**
- **Financial aid**
- **Summing it up**

REQUIREMENTS FOR ADMISSION

Each college/school of pharmacy has its own admissions requirements and deadlines. Contact the institution you are considering to determine its exact requirements.

Typically, each college/school requires a minimum of two years pre-pharmacy, three letters of reference, transcripts, a personal interview, and a minimum score on the PCAT. Please note that some schools of pharmacy now require three years of pre-pharmacy, and at least one school requires a B.S. degree to be considered for admission.

The PCAT

If the college/school you are applying to requires the PCAT, you should take it in the fall before you apply. This gives you the opportunity to retake the PCAT in the winter, if needed. Note that many colleges/schools of pharmacy do not penalize applicants for taking the test more than once, and you can often use your highest score. Because PCAT requirements vary at each college/school, be sure to check with individual testing guidelines. You can usually take the PCAT until you receive a score that is above the minimum requirement of the institution to which you are applying.

chapter 4

HEALTH PROFESSION ADVISERS

Most colleges have health profession advisers who can assist in determining the courses that satisfy the requirements for admission to your school(s) of choice. If you are enrolled in an institution that does not have a college of pharmacy, you should seek advice from your health profession and pre-pharmacy advisers. For more information on health advisers, contact the National Association of Advisers for the Health Professions (NAAHP), P.O. Box 1518, Champaign, IL 61824-1518; Phone: (217) 355-0063; Fax: (217) 355-1287; E-mail: NAAHP@aol.com; Web site: www.naahp.org.

APPLICATION PROCESS

The following steps should be considered when applying to a college of pharmacy:

1. Meet with or call the admissions officer to determine the requirements for admission.

2. Be sure that you meet the pre-pharmacy requirements of the college/school or that you are on track to meet the requirements.

3. Make certain that your current transcripts are in order and that they are sent to the college by your registrar's office. Note: Be sure to update your transcript as you finish requirements because you will most likely have at least one semester of grades that are not on the submitted transcript.

4. Be sure that your preprofessional evaluations have been submitted to your home institution (this is done by your faculty adviser, pre-health adviser, or, in some institutions, by a professor in your major).

Letters of Recommendation

TIP

Do not submit letters from clergy or from political contacts unless the political contact is a relative or pharmacist.

Letters from employers are preferred to determine your work ethic. Letters from professors are also desirable. If one professor is already involved in the pre-professional evaluation, other professors or employers should be used. For example, if you have worked for a pharmacist or have a pharmacist who knows you well (i.e., is familiar with your academic status and work ethic), use this professional as a reference.

PharmCAS—Pharmacy College Application Service

PharmCAS is a centralized application service designed to facilitate application to the colleges/schools of pharmacy in the United States. Students complete a single application and supply one complete set of transcripts (official transcripts from college[s] attended) and can apply to multiple Pharm.D. programs. PharmCAS processes the applications for those schools that participate in the program. Interested students should log on to www.pharmcas.org for more information.

Interviews

Many colleges/schools of pharmacy require interviews with students. These interviews are granted based on your PCAT scores and grade point average.

For your interview, you should:

1 Dress in business attire.

2 Be prepared to write a one-page essay (some schools require this, but not all).

3 Be honest and clear on why you want to enter the pharmacy profession.

4 Show that you are animated and excited about the profession.

5 Be prepared to discuss any issues in your academic background that would raise questions with the admissions committee.

6 Expect questions about your interests and your strengths and weaknesses.

7 Make consistent eye contact with your interviewer.

PHARMACY EDUCATION COSTS

The following is an example of the costs incurred by a pharmacy student entering the University of Tennessee College of Pharmacy. These costs are for the 2005–06 academic year.

Costs per academic year	First year	Second year	Third year	Fourth year
Tuition & fees (Resident)	$12,960	$12,787	$12,787	$12,787
Tuition & fees (Nonresident)	$25,460	$25,287	$25,287	$25,287
Books & supplies	$2,874	$905	$535	$260
Living expenses	$11,786	$14,738	$16,198	$16,213
TOTAL (Resident)	**$27,620**	**$28,430**	**$29,520**	**$29,260**
TOTAL (Nonresident)	**$40,120**	**$40,930**	**$42,020**	**$41,760**

FINANCIAL AID

There is a variety of financial aid available for students entering pharmacy programs. You may, for instance, be eligible for one or more of the following federal aid programs:

- Pell Grants (federal funding available for students on a needs basis)
- Federal Work Study (federal and local funds available to pay salaries for students working on campus)
- Supplemental Educational Opportunity Grants (SEOG)
- Health Professions Student Loans (HPSL)
- Health Education Assistance Loans (HEAL)
- Veterans' benefits
- National Direct Student Loan Programs
- Family Education Loans

For more information about eligibility and how to apply, call the Federal Student Aid Information Center at (800) 4-FED-AID.

In addition to federal programs, most colleges/schools of pharmacy offer need-based and/or merit scholarships to students. Each college or school also has its own financial aid program and may offer loans, grants, and scholarships. You should request financial aid information from each of the pharmacy programs to which you apply.

Many private foundations and organizations also have scholarship programs. Most libraries have directories listing foundations and other private grants to individuals. One such directory is *Peterson's Scholarships, Grants & Prizes*, which can be purchased at bookstores or online at www.petersons.com. Libraries also carry reference volumes that describe in detail all forms and sources of financial aid for undergraduate, professional, and graduate study.

SUMMING IT UP

- Each college or school of pharmacy has its own admission requirements and deadlines. Contact the institution you are considering for exact requirements.

- Typically, each college or school of pharmacy requires a minimum of two years of pre-pharmacy education, three letters of recommendation, transcripts, a personal interview, and a minimum score on the PCAT.

- The Pharmacy College Application Service (PharmCAS) is a centralized online application service at www.pharmcas.org designed to facilitate application to colleges or schools of pharmacy.

Postgraduate Education

OVERVIEW

- **Residencies**
- **Frequently asked questions about pharmacy residencies**
- **Fellowships**
- **Graduate education**
- **Summing it up**

RESIDENCIES

In 1953, the American Society of Health-Systems Pharmacists (ASHP) began the accreditation of postgraduate training programs in hospital pharmacy. These programs were called hospital pharmacy residencies. During the past twenty years, residency programs have proliferated. The ASHP is the accrediting body for hospital pharmacy residencies, as well as specialty residencies. There are more than 200 accredited residency programs in the United States, as well as other nonaccredited fellowship, residency, and specialty residency programs. This number is growing every year.

FREQUENTLY ASKED QUESTIONS ABOUT PHARMACY RESIDENCIES*

What is a pharmacy residency?

A pharmacy residency is an organized, directed postgraduate learning experience in a defined area of pharmacy practice.

What types of pharmacy residencies are there?

The most common type of residency is a pharmacy practice residency, conducted in an institution under the preceptorship of the director of the pharmacy

---

* From the ASHP publication "What Is a Pharmacy Residency?" Reprinted with permission of the American Society of Health-Systems Pharmacists.

department. The objective of residency training in pharmacy practice is to develop competent practitioners who are able to provide a broad scope of pharmaceutical services (clinical, informational, drug distribution, product formulation, quality control, supportive administrative, etc.). Training typically involves structured rotations within the pharmacy department and within other departments in the hospital and includes participation in conferences, seminars, research projects, and related activities. Many residencies also provide limited experience in other hospital pharmacies or organized health-care settings.

Another type of residency is a specialty pharmacy practice area. It emphasizes the provision of pharmaceutical care to a variety of patients. Although most of the resident's training occurs in an institution, less emphasis is placed on the overall operation of a pharmacy department. Most specialty residencies are available only to those who have completed the Pharm.D. degree. These specialty residencies include psychiatry, drug information, pharmacokinetics, cardiology, geriatrics, pediatrics, nutrition, critical care, etc.

What is meant by an "accredited" residency?

The ASHP is the accrediting body for the types of residencies described. The ASHP grants accreditation to institutions that meet certain standards of practice and demonstrate a quality training program. Accreditation of a pharmacy residency program provides assurance to prospective residents that the program has met the basic requirements and is therefore an acceptable site for postgraduate training in pharmacy practice.

How many hours are required to complete a pharmacy residency?

A minimum of 2,000 hours of training extending over a minimum of fifty weeks is required in an ASHP-accredited residency program—the equivalent of one average work year. Some residency programs are offered only in conjunction with an advanced degree (M.S. or Pharm.D.) in a college of pharmacy or graduate school. Such programs are commonly referred to as "affiliated" residencies and generally require two years for completion. Residents in some affiliated programs pursue the residency part-time so there will be adequate time for course work, thesis research, and other degree requirements. Many affiliated programs, however, allow the residency to be taken either before or after the postgraduate academic course work.

Other residency programs ("nonaffiliated" residencies) are offered independently of an advanced degree and typically require one year of full-time work for completion. An applicant who already holds an advanced degree would normally choose one of these programs if he or she is interested in pursuing residency training.

Do residents earn a salary?

All accredited residency programs provide the resident with a stipend, although the amount varies from program to program, depending on the number of actual residency training hours per year, the value of any fringe benefits provided, and geographic location (cost of living). The stipends are generally inadequate to cover living costs for a resident having significant family support responsibilities. Furthermore, a residency, whether affiliated or not, requires a full-time commitment on the part of the resident and usually does not permit supplementing income through part-time employment. Therefore, applicants with family support obligations should have financial resources in addition to the residency stipend on which they can rely during the residency training period.

Who should consider taking an accredited pharmacy residency?

Any pharmacist or pharmacy student whose career objectives center around institutional or clinical pharmacy practice should give serious consideration to residency training. Because of the concentrated nature of the training in a residency program, an individual may develop competence in a broader scope of pharmacy practice in a one- or two-year residency program than might be expected from several years as a staff pharmacist with a fixed assignment. Many "positions available" listings in the ASHP Personnel Placement Service specify completion of an accredited residency as an employment prerequisite.

What are the requirements for admission to an accredited pharmacy residency?

An applicant must be a graduate of an ACPE-accredited college of pharmacy (or must have graduated before the beginning date of the residency) and should have demonstrated an interest in and aptitude for advanced training in pharmacy. Some residencies require that the applicant be licensed to practice before entering the program, although others will accept applicants who have some limited internship obligation remaining for completion of state board licensure requirements. In the case of an affiliated residency program, the applicant must satisfy both the requirements of the college of pharmacy or graduate school for admission to the advanced degree program and the requirements established by the institution in which the residency is offered. Residents in ASHP-accredited programs should be members of the American Society of Health-Systems Pharmacists. Students with B.S. or Pharm.D. degrees who are applying for postgraduate residency and/or fellowship programs should write to the American Society of Health-Systems Pharmacists Residency Matching Program, 7272 Wisconsin Avenue, Bethesda, MD 20814; Phone: (301) 657-3000; Fax: (301) 652-8278; Web site: www.ashp.org. A list of accredited residencies may be obtained from the ASHP.

NOTE

The average salary for residents in 2002–2003 was $34,000 per year.

FELLOWSHIPS

Fellowships focus on research in a specific area and usually require the completion of a residency. They are typically two years long and are designed to prepare the fellow for a career in education or industry.

For more information contact:

The American College of Clinical Pharmacy
3101 Broadway, Suite 650
Kansas City, MO 64111
Phone: (816) 531-2177
Fax: (816) 531-4990
E-mail: accp@accp.com
Web site: www.accp.com

GRADUATE EDUCATION

Graduate education in colleges of pharmacy can be broadly divided into two areas:

1. *Pharmaceutical Sciences:* This includes medicinal chemistry, pharmaceutics, pharmacokinetics, drug metabolism, pharmacology, and toxicology. M.S. and Ph.D. degrees are offered.

2. *Health Science Administration:* This area includes pharmacoeconomics, health policy, administration, practice management, and social and administrative science programs. M.S. and Ph.D. degrees are offered.

For more information contact:

The American Association of Colleges of Pharmacy
1426 Prince Street
Alexandria, VA 22314
Phone: (703) 739-2330
Fax: (703) 836-8982
E-mail: mail@accp.org
Web site: www.aacp.org

SUMMING IT UP

- Postgraduate education is comprised of accredited and nonaccredited residencies, fellowships, and graduate education.

- A residency is an organized, directed postgraduate learning experience in a defined area of pharmacy practice.

- A minimum of 2,000 hours of training conducted over 50 weeks is required as part of an American Society of Health-Systems Pharmacy (ASHP)–accredited residency program.

- Fellowships focus on research in a specific area and usually require the completion of a residency.

- Graduate education in colleges or schools of pharmacy can be divided into two broad categories: pharmaceutical sciences and health science administration.

Making Pharmacy Your Career

chapter 6

OVERVIEW

- **Career opportunities**
- **Pharmacist responsibilities for patient-centered pharmaceutical care**
- **Factors affecting the pharmacy profession**
- **Summing it up**

CAREER OPPORTUNITIES

Since the 1960s, pharmacy education and practice have undergone incredible changes—changes that continue into the twenty-first century. Pharmacy, an old and honored profession, is still evolving. Job opportunities are available in several areas, including, but not limited to:

- Community pharmacy (independent practice or chain store)
- Hospital pharmacy
- Pharmaceutical industry
- Government
- Geriatric pharmacy
- Pediatrics and other clinical practice areas
- Veterinary pharmacy
- Compounding
- Home infusion

Current job opportunities also include clinical practice in a variety of specialty areas, including nuclear pharmacy, pharmacotherapy, nutrition support practice, psychiatric practice, and oncology practice. These areas are recognized by the Board of Pharmaceutical Specialties. In addition, practice in managed care is still evolving, and there will be opportunities in areas not yet identified.

Educational opportunities beyond the pharmacy degree include graduate education in the pharmaceutical or medical sciences, including medicine and dentistry. There is also the opportunity to further one's education in a collateral area by combining a pharmacy career with a law degree or M.B.A., for example.

Individuals who earn a pharmacy degree have many opportunities available to them. Postgraduate education also offers an excellent opportunity for building on the basic pharmacy education.

The following are brief descriptions of some of the career opportunities available when the basic requirements for pharmacy licensure are completed.

Community/Ambulatory Practice

Community pharmacists are becoming practitioners who provide a variety of health-care services to patients by dispensing medications; providing patient education on disease and medications; and performing immunizations, allergy shots, and therapeutic drug monitoring. In addition to these responsibilities, pharmacists are also responsible for educating the patient about his/her medications.

Because of the ever-increasing quantity of pharmaceutical knowledge, professionals in other health-care areas turn more frequently to pharmacists for advice and assistance. For instance, pharmacists may contribute information on selecting the best drug therapy for a patient and help physicians monitor a patient's progress. Pharmacists must detect possible adverse reactions as a result of drug-drug, drug-food, and drug-disease interactions. They also have the responsibility of advising patients in the use of nonprescription drugs. In addition, they must make recommendations to patients and other health professionals for avoiding problems with drug use.

The practice of community pharmacy is also a business. In addition to patient-care activities, pharmacists must also manage people, resources, and time. The opportunity for community involvement and the respect of the patient make community practice exciting. Opportunities are available in rural and metropolitan areas, as well as several settings, such as apothecaries, chain drug stores, and independent community pharmacies.

For more information about community/ambulatory practice, contact the American Pharmaceutical Association (APhA), 2215 Constitution Avenue NW, Washington, D.C. 20037-2985; Phone: (202) 628-4410; Fax: (202) 783-2351; Web site: www.aphanet.org.

Institutional Pharmacy

Pharmacists in institutions supervise the distribution of drugs to patients and provide therapeutic drug monitoring, formulary services, drug information services, and management services. In addition, pharmacists are assuming greater responsibility for patient education. This includes taking medication histories of admitted patients; monitoring drug therapies; managing the drug regimens of patients; and making patient rounds with physicians and nurses to provide drug information, participate in cardiac codes, and provide pharmacokinetic and therapeutic consultations to physicians, physician's assistants, and advanced practice nurses.

Pharmacists serve as consultants to other health professionals on drug therapy and conduct in-service education programs for them. In addition, some pharmacists may work in a nuclear pharmacy, preparing various radioactive testing agents, as well as radio pharmaceuticals used in chemotherapy regimens for patients with cancer.

Decentralization of pharmacy services has expanded institutional pharmacy to a more clinical role. Institutional pharmacists now specialize in a variety of areas, including practice management, critical care, ambulatory care, geriatrics, pediatrics, medicine, surgery, oncology, psychiatry, nutrition support, and drug education.

For more information about institutional pharmacy practice, contact the American Society of Health-Systems Pharmacists (ASHP), 7272 Wisconsin Avenue, Bethesda, MD 20814; Phone: (301) 657-3000; Fax: (301) 652-8278; Web site: www.ashp.org.

Pharmaceutical Industry

Many pharmaceutical firms employ pharmacists in clinical research, product development, quality control, sales, marketing, management, and several other roles. Pharmacists, as well as other scientists, are responsible for testing and controlling the production of drugs. Once pharmaceuticals have been manufactured, they must be marketed. Pharmacists work in regulatory affairs, dealing with the Food and Drug Administration (FDA), as well as in professional affairs. The professional affairs area includes working with other pharmacists, physicians, and health-care providers, as well as with the general public.

Pharmacists also serve as medical service representatives—the sales force of the pharmaceutical industry. These representatives call on physicians, dentists, veterinarians, pharmacists (hospital, community, extended-care facilities, and government agencies), and nurses to explain the uses and merits of the products that their firms manufacture. In addition, the clinical research area uses pharmacists to monitor and control field research and to select research sites.

Another area of the pharmaceutical industry is product and consumer information. Pharmacists in this field provide product information to health-care providers and to the public. They also serve as a resource for sales and marketing forces. For more information on opportunities in the pharmaceutical industry, contact The Pharmaceutical Research and Manufacturers of America (PhRMA); 1100 15th Street NW, Washington, D.C. 20005; Phone: (202) 835-3400; Fax: (202) 835-3414; Web site: www.phrma.org.

Government Pharmacy Practice

Many pharmacists work for public-health departments on a federal, state, or local level. In the FDA, pharmacists work with physicians and other health-care providers in assessing sound manufacturing practices and the efficacy of new drug products. In the U.S. Public Health Service, pharmacists are employed as institutional pharmacy practi-

NOTE

Clinical practice has changed the role of the pharmacist to that of a provider of pharmaceutical care.

tioners, administrators, or clinical pharmacists. Pharmacy positions are also available in other government agencies, such as the National Institutes of Health, where practitioners provide patient-centered pharmaceutical care and conduct research.

Pharmacists may participate at the local or state government level as members of licensing boards (State Boards of Pharmacy) as administrators, inspectors, or board members. Pharmaceutical services are also provided in health-care facilities on military bases in the United States and abroad.

Nuclear Pharmacy

Individuals who specialize in nuclear pharmacy work with and prepare radioactive medications (diagnostic or therapeutic agents). Pharmacists must be certified to work with radioactive materials; generally, a postgraduate course is required. Pharmacy students may take electives in nuclear pharmacy in schools of pharmacy that offer such programs. Postgraduate courses may cover the minimum requirement of 2,000 hours of work or may include graduate course work leading to an M.S. degree or Ph.D. Nuclear Pharmacy was the first board-certified specialty recognized by the Board of Pharmaceutical Specialties.

For more information on nuclear pharmacy and other areas of specialization, contact: Board of Pharmaceutical Specialties (BPS), 2215 Constitution Avenue NW, Washington, D.C. 20037-2985; Phone: (202) 429-7591; Fax: (202) 429-6304; E-mail: bps@aphanet.org; Web site: www.bpsweb.org.

Geriatric Pharmacy Practice

The fastest growing segment of the population consists of individuals over the age of 65. In 1880, this group represented 3 percent of the population, whereas in 1980 it represented 11.3 percent of the population. It is estimated that by 2010, 22.5 percent of the population will be over the age of 65.

Geriatric patients have more chronic diseases and, therefore, use more over-the-counter prescription medications than any other age group. Because of their unique needs and the unique problems of drug therapy for the elderly, a specialty in geriatric pharmacy practice developed. The geriatric pharmacist provides therapeutic consultation, patient counseling and education, in-service education to nursing staffs of extended-care facilities, and therapeutic consultations with physicians on the drug therapy regimens of the elderly. In addition, dispensing services are also required for these facilities. This new area of practice offers a rewarding and challenging career.

For more information on geriatric pharmacy or consultant practice, contact: American Society of Consultant Pharmacists, 1321 Duke Street, Alexandria, VA 22314-3563; Phone: (703) 739-1300; Fax: (703) 739-1321; E-mail: info@ascp.com; Web site: www.ascp.com.

Clinical Practice Specialty Areas

During the past twenty years, a clinical practice of pharmacy developed that focused on the provision of rational therapeutics to patients in specific areas. For example, there are pharmacists who now practice in specialty areas such as pediatrics, oncology, psychiatry, critical-care medicine, pharmacokinetics, geriatrics, pulmonary medicine, and infectious diseases. These practitioners provide services to patients in hospitals and/or clinics.

The majority of these practitioners today have a Pharm.D. degree and either a specialty residency or a fellowship. Specialties that are recognized for board certification by the Board of Pharmaceutical Specialties include nutrition support pharmacy, pharmacotherapy, psychiatry pharmacy, and oncology pharmacy.

For more information on board certification of pharmacists, contact: Board of Pharmaceutical Specialties (BPS), 2215 Constitution Avenue NW, Washington, D.C. 20037-2985; Phone: (202) 429-7591; Fax: (202) 429-6304; E-mail: bps@aphanet.org; Web site: www.bpsweb.org.

For more information on specialty clinical practice areas, contact: American College of Clinical Pharmacy (ACCP), 3101 Broadway, Suite 650, Kansas City, MO 64111; Phone: (816) 531-2177; Fax: (816) 531-4990; E-mail: accp@accp.com; Web site: www.accp.com.

PHARMACIST RESPONSIBILITIES FOR PATIENT-CENTERED PHARMACEUTICAL CARE

1 *Patient education*—Discuss the correct way for patients to take medication; educate patients about disease; and answer questions about drug therapy, drug interactions, and issues such as diet and exercise.

2 *Monitoring*—Monitor patients' therapy to ensure that their medications are working effectively, with no side effects or adverse drug reactions (ADR). Assess patients' understanding of disease and drug therapy in order to improve patient compliance/adherence.

3 *Providing pharmacokinetic consultations*—Provide information to physicians on drug absorption, drug excretion, and drug metabolism of specific drugs, allowing for individualized dosing and ensuring optimal drug therapy results.

4 *Relating drug information*—Provide information to physicians, nurses, dentists, and other health-care providers, as well as to the public.

NOTE

In the future, a residency or fellowship will be required in addition to the basic Pharm.D. degree to practice in specialty areas.

⑤ *Prescribing*—Pharmacists have traditionally been responsible for recommending over-the-counter drugs to patients. However, during the past several years, there have been changes in pharmacy practice laws in several states. These changes provide for pharmacists prescribing under protocol and also for collaborative-care agreements between pharmacists and physicians, as well as other health-care providers.

⑥ *Disease management*—Work in concert with other health-care professionals to provide disease management for specific patient populations. For example, diabetes and asthma are two chronic diseases with which pharmacists have been actively involved as members of the disease management team.

FACTORS AFFECTING THE PHARMACY PROFESSION

There are both internal and external factors that affect the future of the pharmacy profession. The following factors have impacted the pharmacy profession.

❶ *Federal Legislation:* For example, the Health Insurance Portability Accountability Act (HIPAA) has had a significant effect on the functioning of all health-care professionals, including pharmacists. HIPAA primarily affects the record-keeping systems in pharmacies and the patient's right to privacy. Other legislation, such as the prescription drug benefit for Medicare patients, also plays a major role in pharmacy.

❷ *Aging U.S. Population:* As a greater percentage of U.S. citizens exceed 65 years of age, the demand for pharmacy services will grow as the number of prescriptions dispensed increases. By 2006, it is projected that more than 4.4 billion prescriptions will be dispensed, creating a greater demand for pharmacists.

❸ *Corporate Mergers:* Corporate mergers have impacted both the pharmaceutical industry, as well as the hospital and chain drug industries.

❹ *Automation/Technology:* As automation and technology advance, the pharmacist's ability to provide better patient care will be enhanced.

❺ *Drug Development:* New medications mean better treatments for patients, resulting in a greater need for pharmacists to provide new drug information to patients and health-care providers.

❻ *Staffing:* There is a shortage of pharmacists, nurses, allied health professionals, and, in some locations, dentists and medical specialists. As a result, the starting salaries of pharmacists have increased dramatically during the past four years. In 2004, the average starting salary for graduates in the Southeast exceeded $88,000.

The pharmacy profession is dynamic and ever-changing. If you select pharmacy as your career goal, you will find it rewarding and challenging. Contact a college/school of pharmacy or your state pharmacy association for more information on pharmacy career opportunities and pharmacy education.

SUMMING IT UP

- In addition to the more traditional careers in pharmacy, opportunities abound in a variety of specialty areas including nuclear pharmacy, pharmacotherapy, nutrition support practice, psychiatry, and oncology.

- Pharmacists are now responsible for patient-centered pharmaceutical care in the areas of patient education, monitoring, pharmacokinetic consultation, drug information, prescribing, and disease management.

PART IV

PRACTICE TEST

PRACTICE TEST 2

PRACTICE TEST 2 ANSWER SHEET

Reading Comprehension

1. Ⓐ Ⓑ Ⓒ Ⓓ   11. Ⓐ Ⓑ Ⓒ Ⓓ   21. Ⓐ Ⓑ Ⓒ Ⓓ   31. Ⓐ Ⓑ Ⓒ Ⓓ   41. Ⓐ Ⓑ Ⓒ Ⓓ
2. Ⓐ Ⓑ Ⓒ Ⓓ   12. Ⓐ Ⓑ Ⓒ Ⓓ   22. Ⓐ Ⓑ Ⓒ Ⓓ   32. Ⓐ Ⓑ Ⓒ Ⓓ   42. Ⓐ Ⓑ Ⓒ Ⓓ
3. Ⓐ Ⓑ Ⓒ Ⓓ   13. Ⓐ Ⓑ Ⓒ Ⓓ   23. Ⓐ Ⓑ Ⓒ Ⓓ   33. Ⓐ Ⓑ Ⓒ Ⓓ   43. Ⓐ Ⓑ Ⓒ Ⓓ
4. Ⓐ Ⓑ Ⓒ Ⓓ   14. Ⓐ Ⓑ Ⓒ Ⓓ   24. Ⓐ Ⓑ Ⓒ Ⓓ   34. Ⓐ Ⓑ Ⓒ Ⓓ   44. Ⓐ Ⓑ Ⓒ Ⓓ
5. Ⓐ Ⓑ Ⓒ Ⓓ   15. Ⓐ Ⓑ Ⓒ Ⓓ   25. Ⓐ Ⓑ Ⓒ Ⓓ   35. Ⓐ Ⓑ Ⓒ Ⓓ   45. Ⓐ Ⓑ Ⓒ Ⓓ
6. Ⓐ Ⓑ Ⓒ Ⓓ   16. Ⓐ Ⓑ Ⓒ Ⓓ   26. Ⓐ Ⓑ Ⓒ Ⓓ   36. Ⓐ Ⓑ Ⓒ Ⓓ   46. Ⓐ Ⓑ Ⓒ Ⓓ
7. Ⓐ Ⓑ Ⓒ Ⓓ   17. Ⓐ Ⓑ Ⓒ Ⓓ   27. Ⓐ Ⓑ Ⓒ Ⓓ   37. Ⓐ Ⓑ Ⓒ Ⓓ   47. Ⓐ Ⓑ Ⓒ Ⓓ
8. Ⓐ Ⓑ Ⓒ Ⓓ   18. Ⓐ Ⓑ Ⓒ Ⓓ   28. Ⓐ Ⓑ Ⓒ Ⓓ   38. Ⓐ Ⓑ Ⓒ Ⓓ   48. Ⓐ Ⓑ Ⓒ Ⓓ
9. Ⓐ Ⓑ Ⓒ Ⓓ   19. Ⓐ Ⓑ Ⓒ Ⓓ   29. Ⓐ Ⓑ Ⓒ Ⓓ   39. Ⓐ Ⓑ Ⓒ Ⓓ
10. Ⓐ Ⓑ Ⓒ Ⓓ   20. Ⓐ Ⓑ Ⓒ Ⓓ   30. Ⓐ Ⓑ Ⓒ Ⓓ   40. Ⓐ Ⓑ Ⓒ Ⓓ

Biology

1. Ⓐ Ⓑ Ⓒ Ⓓ   13. Ⓐ Ⓑ Ⓒ Ⓓ   25. Ⓐ Ⓑ Ⓒ Ⓓ   37. Ⓐ Ⓑ Ⓒ Ⓓ   49. Ⓐ Ⓑ Ⓒ Ⓓ
2. Ⓐ Ⓑ Ⓒ Ⓓ   14. Ⓐ Ⓑ Ⓒ Ⓓ   26. Ⓐ Ⓑ Ⓒ Ⓓ   38. Ⓐ Ⓑ Ⓒ Ⓓ   50. Ⓐ Ⓑ Ⓒ Ⓓ
3. Ⓐ Ⓑ Ⓒ Ⓓ   15. Ⓐ Ⓑ Ⓒ Ⓓ   27. Ⓐ Ⓑ Ⓒ Ⓓ   39. Ⓐ Ⓑ Ⓒ Ⓓ   51. Ⓐ Ⓑ Ⓒ Ⓓ
4. Ⓐ Ⓑ Ⓒ Ⓓ   16. Ⓐ Ⓑ Ⓒ Ⓓ   28. Ⓐ Ⓑ Ⓒ Ⓓ   40. Ⓐ Ⓑ Ⓒ Ⓓ   52. Ⓐ Ⓑ Ⓒ Ⓓ
5. Ⓐ Ⓑ Ⓒ Ⓓ   17. Ⓐ Ⓑ Ⓒ Ⓓ   29. Ⓐ Ⓑ Ⓒ Ⓓ   41. Ⓐ Ⓑ Ⓒ Ⓓ   53. Ⓐ Ⓑ Ⓒ Ⓓ
6. Ⓐ Ⓑ Ⓒ Ⓓ   18. Ⓐ Ⓑ Ⓒ Ⓓ   30. Ⓐ Ⓑ Ⓒ Ⓓ   42. Ⓐ Ⓑ Ⓒ Ⓓ   54. Ⓐ Ⓑ Ⓒ Ⓓ
7. Ⓐ Ⓑ Ⓒ Ⓓ   19. Ⓐ Ⓑ Ⓒ Ⓓ   31. Ⓐ Ⓑ Ⓒ Ⓓ   43. Ⓐ Ⓑ Ⓒ Ⓓ   55. Ⓐ Ⓑ Ⓒ Ⓓ
8. Ⓐ Ⓑ Ⓒ Ⓓ   20. Ⓐ Ⓑ Ⓒ Ⓓ   32. Ⓐ Ⓑ Ⓒ Ⓓ   44. Ⓐ Ⓑ Ⓒ Ⓓ   56. Ⓐ Ⓑ Ⓒ Ⓓ
9. Ⓐ Ⓑ Ⓒ Ⓓ   21. Ⓐ Ⓑ Ⓒ Ⓓ   33. Ⓐ Ⓑ Ⓒ Ⓓ   45. Ⓐ Ⓑ Ⓒ Ⓓ   57. Ⓐ Ⓑ Ⓒ Ⓓ
10. Ⓐ Ⓑ Ⓒ Ⓓ   22. Ⓐ Ⓑ Ⓒ Ⓓ   34. Ⓐ Ⓑ Ⓒ Ⓓ   46. Ⓐ Ⓑ Ⓒ Ⓓ   58. Ⓐ Ⓑ Ⓒ Ⓓ
11. Ⓐ Ⓑ Ⓒ Ⓓ   23. Ⓐ Ⓑ Ⓒ Ⓓ   35. Ⓐ Ⓑ Ⓒ Ⓓ   47. Ⓐ Ⓑ Ⓒ Ⓓ
12. Ⓐ Ⓑ Ⓒ Ⓓ   24. Ⓐ Ⓑ Ⓒ Ⓓ   36. Ⓐ Ⓑ Ⓒ Ⓓ   48. Ⓐ Ⓑ Ⓒ Ⓓ

answer sheet

Quantitative Ability

1. Ⓐ Ⓑ Ⓒ Ⓓ	13. Ⓐ Ⓑ Ⓒ Ⓓ	25. Ⓐ Ⓑ Ⓒ Ⓓ	37. Ⓐ Ⓑ Ⓒ Ⓓ	49. Ⓐ Ⓑ Ⓒ Ⓓ
2. Ⓐ Ⓑ Ⓒ Ⓓ	14. Ⓐ Ⓑ Ⓒ Ⓓ	26. Ⓐ Ⓑ Ⓒ Ⓓ	38. Ⓐ Ⓑ Ⓒ Ⓓ	50. Ⓐ Ⓑ Ⓒ Ⓓ
3. Ⓐ Ⓑ Ⓒ Ⓓ	15. Ⓐ Ⓑ Ⓒ Ⓓ	27. Ⓐ Ⓑ Ⓒ Ⓓ	39. Ⓐ Ⓑ Ⓒ Ⓓ	51. Ⓐ Ⓑ Ⓒ Ⓓ
4. Ⓐ Ⓑ Ⓒ Ⓓ	16. Ⓐ Ⓑ Ⓒ Ⓓ	28. Ⓐ Ⓑ Ⓒ Ⓓ	40. Ⓐ Ⓑ Ⓒ Ⓓ	52. Ⓐ Ⓑ Ⓒ Ⓓ
5. Ⓐ Ⓑ Ⓒ Ⓓ	17. Ⓐ Ⓑ Ⓒ Ⓓ	29. Ⓐ Ⓑ Ⓒ Ⓓ	41. Ⓐ Ⓑ Ⓒ Ⓓ	53. Ⓐ Ⓑ Ⓒ Ⓓ
6. Ⓐ Ⓑ Ⓒ Ⓓ	18. Ⓐ Ⓑ Ⓒ Ⓓ	30. Ⓐ Ⓑ Ⓒ Ⓓ	42. Ⓐ Ⓑ Ⓒ Ⓓ	54. Ⓐ Ⓑ Ⓒ Ⓓ
7. Ⓐ Ⓑ Ⓒ Ⓓ	19. Ⓐ Ⓑ Ⓒ Ⓓ	31. Ⓐ Ⓑ Ⓒ Ⓓ	43. Ⓐ Ⓑ Ⓒ Ⓓ	55. Ⓐ Ⓑ Ⓒ Ⓓ
8. Ⓐ Ⓑ Ⓒ Ⓓ	20. Ⓐ Ⓑ Ⓒ Ⓓ	32. Ⓐ Ⓑ Ⓒ Ⓓ	44. Ⓐ Ⓑ Ⓒ Ⓓ	56. Ⓐ Ⓑ Ⓒ Ⓓ
9. Ⓐ Ⓑ Ⓒ Ⓓ	21. Ⓐ Ⓑ Ⓒ Ⓓ	33. Ⓐ Ⓑ Ⓒ Ⓓ	45. Ⓐ Ⓑ Ⓒ Ⓓ	57. Ⓐ Ⓑ Ⓒ Ⓓ
10. Ⓐ Ⓑ Ⓒ Ⓓ	22. Ⓐ Ⓑ Ⓒ Ⓓ	34. Ⓐ Ⓑ Ⓒ Ⓓ	46. Ⓐ Ⓑ Ⓒ Ⓓ	58. Ⓐ Ⓑ Ⓒ Ⓓ
11. Ⓐ Ⓑ Ⓒ Ⓓ	23. Ⓐ Ⓑ Ⓒ Ⓓ	35. Ⓐ Ⓑ Ⓒ Ⓓ	47. Ⓐ Ⓑ Ⓒ Ⓓ	
12. Ⓐ Ⓑ Ⓒ Ⓓ	24. Ⓐ Ⓑ Ⓒ Ⓓ	36. Ⓐ Ⓑ Ⓒ Ⓓ	48. Ⓐ Ⓑ Ⓒ Ⓓ	

Chemistry

1. Ⓐ Ⓑ Ⓒ Ⓓ	13. Ⓐ Ⓑ Ⓒ Ⓓ	25. Ⓐ Ⓑ Ⓒ Ⓓ	37. Ⓐ Ⓑ Ⓒ Ⓓ	49. Ⓐ Ⓑ Ⓒ Ⓓ
2. Ⓐ Ⓑ Ⓒ Ⓓ	14. Ⓐ Ⓑ Ⓒ Ⓓ	26. Ⓐ Ⓑ Ⓒ Ⓓ	38. Ⓐ Ⓑ Ⓒ Ⓓ	50. Ⓐ Ⓑ Ⓒ Ⓓ
3. Ⓐ Ⓑ Ⓒ Ⓓ	15. Ⓐ Ⓑ Ⓒ Ⓓ	27. Ⓐ Ⓑ Ⓒ Ⓓ	39. Ⓐ Ⓑ Ⓒ Ⓓ	51. Ⓐ Ⓑ Ⓒ Ⓓ
4. Ⓐ Ⓑ Ⓒ Ⓓ	16. Ⓐ Ⓑ Ⓒ Ⓓ	28. Ⓐ Ⓑ Ⓒ Ⓓ	40. Ⓐ Ⓑ Ⓒ Ⓓ	52. Ⓐ Ⓑ Ⓒ Ⓓ
5. Ⓐ Ⓑ Ⓒ Ⓓ	17. Ⓐ Ⓑ Ⓒ Ⓓ	29. Ⓐ Ⓑ Ⓒ Ⓓ	41. Ⓐ Ⓑ Ⓒ Ⓓ	53. Ⓐ Ⓑ Ⓒ Ⓓ
6. Ⓐ Ⓑ Ⓒ Ⓓ	18. Ⓐ Ⓑ Ⓒ Ⓓ	30. Ⓐ Ⓑ Ⓒ Ⓓ	42. Ⓐ Ⓑ Ⓒ Ⓓ	54. Ⓐ Ⓑ Ⓒ Ⓓ
7. Ⓐ Ⓑ Ⓒ Ⓓ	19. Ⓐ Ⓑ Ⓒ Ⓓ	31. Ⓐ Ⓑ Ⓒ Ⓓ	43. Ⓐ Ⓑ Ⓒ Ⓓ	55. Ⓐ Ⓑ Ⓒ Ⓓ
8. Ⓐ Ⓑ Ⓒ Ⓓ	20. Ⓐ Ⓑ Ⓒ Ⓓ	32. Ⓐ Ⓑ Ⓒ Ⓓ	44. Ⓐ Ⓑ Ⓒ Ⓓ	56. Ⓐ Ⓑ Ⓒ Ⓓ
9. Ⓐ Ⓑ Ⓒ Ⓓ	21. Ⓐ Ⓑ Ⓒ Ⓓ	33. Ⓐ Ⓑ Ⓒ Ⓓ	45. Ⓐ Ⓑ Ⓒ Ⓓ	57. Ⓐ Ⓑ Ⓒ Ⓓ
10. Ⓐ Ⓑ Ⓒ Ⓓ	22. Ⓐ Ⓑ Ⓒ Ⓓ	34. Ⓐ Ⓑ Ⓒ Ⓓ	46. Ⓐ Ⓑ Ⓒ Ⓓ	58. Ⓐ Ⓑ Ⓒ Ⓓ
11. Ⓐ Ⓑ Ⓒ Ⓓ	23. Ⓐ Ⓑ Ⓒ Ⓓ	35. Ⓐ Ⓑ Ⓒ Ⓓ	47. Ⓐ Ⓑ Ⓒ Ⓓ	
12. Ⓐ Ⓑ Ⓒ Ⓓ	24. Ⓐ Ⓑ Ⓒ Ⓓ	36. Ⓐ Ⓑ Ⓒ Ⓓ	48. Ⓐ Ⓑ Ⓒ Ⓓ	

Verbal Ability

1. Ⓐ Ⓑ Ⓒ Ⓓ   13. Ⓐ Ⓑ Ⓒ Ⓓ   25. Ⓐ Ⓑ Ⓒ Ⓓ   37. Ⓐ Ⓑ Ⓒ Ⓓ   49. Ⓐ Ⓑ Ⓒ Ⓓ

2. Ⓐ Ⓑ Ⓒ Ⓓ   14. Ⓐ Ⓑ Ⓒ Ⓓ   26. Ⓐ Ⓑ Ⓒ Ⓓ   38. Ⓐ Ⓑ Ⓒ Ⓓ   50. Ⓐ Ⓑ Ⓒ Ⓓ

3. Ⓐ Ⓑ Ⓒ Ⓓ   15. Ⓐ Ⓑ Ⓒ Ⓓ   27. Ⓐ Ⓑ Ⓒ Ⓓ   39. Ⓐ Ⓑ Ⓒ Ⓓ   51. Ⓐ Ⓑ Ⓒ Ⓓ

4. Ⓐ Ⓑ Ⓒ Ⓓ   16. Ⓐ Ⓑ Ⓒ Ⓓ   28. Ⓐ Ⓑ Ⓒ Ⓓ   40. Ⓐ Ⓑ Ⓒ Ⓓ   52. Ⓐ Ⓑ Ⓒ Ⓓ

5. Ⓐ Ⓑ Ⓒ Ⓓ   17. Ⓐ Ⓑ Ⓒ Ⓓ   29. Ⓐ Ⓑ Ⓒ Ⓓ   41. Ⓐ Ⓑ Ⓒ Ⓓ   53. Ⓐ Ⓑ Ⓒ Ⓓ

6. Ⓐ Ⓑ Ⓒ Ⓓ   18. Ⓐ Ⓑ Ⓒ Ⓓ   30. Ⓐ Ⓑ Ⓒ Ⓓ   42. Ⓐ Ⓑ Ⓒ Ⓓ   54. Ⓐ Ⓑ Ⓒ Ⓓ

7. Ⓐ Ⓑ Ⓒ Ⓓ   19. Ⓐ Ⓑ Ⓒ Ⓓ   31. Ⓐ Ⓑ Ⓒ Ⓓ   43. Ⓐ Ⓑ Ⓒ Ⓓ   55. Ⓐ Ⓑ Ⓒ Ⓓ

8. Ⓐ Ⓑ Ⓒ Ⓓ   20. Ⓐ Ⓑ Ⓒ Ⓓ   32. Ⓐ Ⓑ Ⓒ Ⓓ   44. Ⓐ Ⓑ Ⓒ Ⓓ   56. Ⓐ Ⓑ Ⓒ Ⓓ

9. Ⓐ Ⓑ Ⓒ Ⓓ   21. Ⓐ Ⓑ Ⓒ Ⓓ   33. Ⓐ Ⓑ Ⓒ Ⓓ   45. Ⓐ Ⓑ Ⓒ Ⓓ   57. Ⓐ Ⓑ Ⓒ Ⓓ

10. Ⓐ Ⓑ Ⓒ Ⓓ   22. Ⓐ Ⓑ Ⓒ Ⓓ   34. Ⓐ Ⓑ Ⓒ Ⓓ   46. Ⓐ Ⓑ Ⓒ Ⓓ   58. Ⓐ Ⓑ Ⓒ Ⓓ

11. Ⓐ Ⓑ Ⓒ Ⓓ   23. Ⓐ Ⓑ Ⓒ Ⓓ   35. Ⓐ Ⓑ Ⓒ Ⓓ   47. Ⓐ Ⓑ Ⓒ Ⓓ

12. Ⓐ Ⓑ Ⓒ Ⓓ   24. Ⓐ Ⓑ Ⓒ Ⓓ   36. Ⓐ Ⓑ Ⓒ Ⓓ   48. Ⓐ Ⓑ Ⓒ Ⓓ

answer sheet

Critical Thinking Essay

48 Questions • 50 Minutes

> **Directions:** Read each of the following six passages and choose the one best answer to the questions that follow each passage.

Anatomy of Swallowing

Dysphagia assumes many forms; the anatomy and mechanics of swallowing demonstrate why. Fifty pairs of muscles
(5) maneuver through a series of voluntary and involuntary neuromuscular contractions as food is chewed and moves from the mouth to the stomach. This process has three distinct phases:

(10) 1. Preparation and oral stage. As food is chewed, the mouth manipulates food and liquid. The tongue propels food and liquid to the back of the mouth, starting the swallowing response.

(15) 2. Oropharyngeal stage. During this stage, food and liquid quickly pass through the pharynx, the canal that connects the mouth to the esophagus. Various muscles steer food or drink to
(20) the esophagus's opening. The larynx, meanwhile, closes tightly and breathing momentarily stops, preventing food and liquid from entering the lungs.

(25) 3. Esophageal stage. The average esophagus is about 9 to 10 inches long and about 1.2 inches wide. Food and liquid pass through the upper esophageal sphincter, a one-way valve to
(30) the esophagus. Peristaltic waves propel food down the esophagus, taking as long as 20 seconds, depending on the food's texture and consistency. When the lower esophageal sphincter
(35) relaxes and the food or liquid enters the stomach, swallowing is complete. While people have some voluntary control over the first stage, the oropha-

ryngeal and esophageal stages occur
(40) involuntarily. A change in any part of these intricate swallowing processes can lead to dysphagia.

Dysphagia Subtypes

The vast majority of disorders occur in
(45) the involuntary stage 2 (oropharyngeal dysphagia) and stage 3 (esophageal dysphagia).

Oropharyngeal dysphagia impairs either food transport to the back of the
(50) mouth or initiation of the swallowing reflex, thus creating a dysfunctional transfer of food and liquid through the pharynx, past the upper esophageal sphincter, and into the esophagus. People
(55) with this type of dysphagia frequently complain that food "sticks" in the throat; they may also choke, cough, or experience nasal regurgitation during swallowing. Oropharyngeal dysphagia is the
(60) most common subtype observed among the elderly, particularly among stroke victims.

Three problems lead to esophageal dysphagia: impaired esophageal peristaltic
(65) motility, esophageal obstruction, and stomach acid reflux into the esophagus. Occasional acid reflux is uncomfortable, but consistent reflux can inflame and narrow the esophagus. Chest discomfort
(70) shortly after swallowing is esophageal dysphagia's hallmark.

Reprinted with permission from *Consultant Pharmacist*, Vol. 18, No. 1, January 2003, Pages 14–15.

1. Which of the following problems does NOT lead to esophageal dysphagia?

   (A) Impaired esophageal peristaltic motility
   (B) Renal obstruction
   (C) Esophageal obstruction
   (D) Stomach acid reflux into the esophagus

2. The average esophagus is approximately

   (A) 2–4 inches long.
   (B) 5–8 inches long.
   (C) 9–10 inches long.
   (D) 11–14 inches long.

3. _____ of muscles maneuver through a series of voluntary and involuntary neuromuscular contractions as food is chewed and moves from the mouth to the stomach.

   (A) Twenty pairs
   (B) Thirty pairs
   (C) Forty pairs
   (D) Fifty pairs

4. The _____ is the canal that connects the mouth to the esophagus.

   (A) pharynx
   (B) canal of Schlemm
   (C) inner canal
   (D) outer canal

5. Dysphagia disorders occur most frequently during which stages of swallowing?

   (A) 1 and 3
   (B) 1 and 4
   (C) 2 and 3
   (D) 1 and 2

6. _____ dysphagia is the most common subtype observed among the elderly, particularly among stroke victims.

   (A) Esophageal
   (B) Oropharyngeal
   (C) Pharyngeal
   (D) Reflux

7. Food and liquid pass through the upper esophageal sphincter, a _____ valve to the esophagus.

   (A) one-way
   (B) two-way
   (C) single
   (D) narrow

8. The _____ closes tightly and breathing momentarily stops, preventing food and liquid from entering the lungs.

   (A) esophagus
   (B) throat
   (C) oropharyngeal canal
   (D) larynx

QUESTIONS 9–18 ARE BASED ON THE FOLLOWING PASSAGE.

Use of Botulinum Toxin Type B for Migraine and Tension Headaches

Headache is the most common patient
(5) complaint reported to health-care professionals. During the past twenty years, there has been heated debate as to whether primary headaches (such as tension headache, migraine headache,
(10) cluster headache, and rebound headache secondary to analgesic abuse) are neurogenic or vascular in origin. Current molecular and functional studies suggest a way of combining both neuro-
(15) logic and vascular causes of headaches.

Botulinum toxin type B, a neurotoxin produced by Clostridium botulinum, acts by blocking acetylcholine release at the neuromuscular junction. Botulinum
(20) toxin type B, unlike botulinum toxin type A, is available as a sterile solution for injection of a purified neurotoxin produced by fermentation of the bacterium. Because of differences in vehicles,
(25) dilution schemes, and laboratory protocols for determining the median lethal dose in mice, units of biological activity of botulinum toxin type B cannot be directly converted into units of activity
(30) of other types of botulinum toxin. However, botulinum toxin type B 5,000 units/ml is generally considered to have a therapeutic effect similar to that of botulinum toxin type A 100 units/ml. There-
(35) fore, botulinum toxin type B may offer benefits to patients for whom we would otherwise use low-dose botulinum toxin type A.

Injectable botulinum toxin type B solu-
(40) tion (Myobloc, South San Francisco, CA) was used at a neurology clinic as an adjunctive therapy for two patients with refractory headaches. One patient had migraine headache and the other,
(45) muscle-tension headache. The frequency of headaches was noted each week after treatment. The severity of headaches was recorded by the patient on a scale from 0–5, where 0 = no headache and
(50) 5 = severe headache, before and after treatment. Botulinum toxin type B was given every three months. The use of prescription pain relievers was also recorded. These two patients were chosen
(55) at random by the neurologist at our neurology clinic to receive botulinum toxin type B.

Reprinted with permission from *American Journal of Health Systems Pharmacist*, Vol. 59, October 1, 2002, Page 1860.

9. What is the trade name of botulinum toxin type B solution?

    (A) Botutoc

    (B) Toxbloc

    (C) Myobloc

    (D) Botubloc

10. The mechanism of action of botulinum toxin type B is to block

    (A) acetylcholine release.

    (B) acetylcholine release at the neuromuscular junction.

    (C) norepinephrine release at the neuromuscular junction.

    (D) choline release at the neuromuscular junction.

11. Which of the following is available in a sterile solution?

(A) Toxin type A

(B) Toxin type B

(C) Toxin type C

(D) Toxin type D

12. According to this passage, what is the most common patient complaint reported to health-care professionals?

(A) Dizziness

(B) Headache

(C) Blurred vision

(D) Dry mouth

13. Which of the following is NOT a reason why botulinum toxin type B cannot be converted into units?

(A) Dilution schemes

(B) Differences in vehicles

(C) Differences in preservatives

(D) Laboratory protocols

14. The scale used in the passage to measure severity of the headache was characterized by

(A) 0 = severe headache.

(B) 5 = severe headache.

(C) 4 = moderate headache.

(D) 3 = not sure.

15. According to the passage, primary headaches include all of the following EXCEPT

(A) tension headache.

(B) cluster headache.

(C) molecular headache.

(D) migraine headache.

16. How often was botulinum toxin type B administered in this study?

(A) Every two months

(B) Every three months

(C) Every four months

(D) Every five months

17. _____ units/ml of botulinum toxin type B are similar to _____ units/ml of botulinum toxin type A.

(A) 2,500; 250

(B) 1,500; 100

(C) 4,000; 100

(D) 5,000; 100

18. According to this passage, Myobloc was used at a _____ clinic.

(A) cardiovascular

(B) surgery

(C) neurology

(D) opthamology

Knocking Down Genes
for Fun and Function

Scientists once thought of eukaryotic RNA as solely active in transcription as
(5) messenger RNA (mRNA), and in translation as transfer RNA (tRNA). After Fire and colleagues first reported that double-stranded RNA (dsRNA) can interfere with gene expression, the con-
(10) ception of how gene transcription works was knocked on its head. Suddenly, these pieces of RNA, which appeared to be cellular detritus sliced out of mRNA, took on importance: They could have a
(15) role in gene suppression.

Subsequent papers by many groups, including these two Hot Papers by Thomas Tuschl and colleagues, formerly of the Max Planck Institute for Biophysi-
(20) cal Chemistry in Gottingen, Germany, clarify how the naturally occurring method of RNA inhibition works, and how engineered small inhibitory RNAs (siRNAs) can be introduced into a cell to
(25) knock down, or suppress, specific gene expression. Barely five years since the concept was first published, researchers are looking to use siRNAs clinically.

The first paper, Tuschl explains, "is the
(30) formal proof that siRNA can do gene silencing." The second paper, he says, shows that siRNAs can direct gene silencing in mammalian cells without interference that kills the cells.
(35) CRUCIAL INFORMATION: In a naturally occurring system, posttranscriptional gene silencing (PTGS) may be a means of protecting cells from transposons or viruses that can produce
(40) dsRNA. Within the cell, these dsRNAs are enzymatically cut into smaller RNA pieces, which then bind to homologous mRNA, preventing translation of certain gene products. RNA fragments
(45) longer than about 30 nucleotides may destroy cellular mRNA, resulting in cytotoxicity and apoptosis.

But Tuschl's group, using a *Drosophila* lysate system, showed that RNAi—the
(50) suppression of gene expression by RNA fragments—occurs when the RNA fragments are 21- or 22-nucleotide duplexes of sense and antisense RNA. These fragments are broken down from the dsRNA
(55) by the Dicer enzyme. Tuschl and colleagues identified efficacious segment lengths for PTGS using synthesized siRNA artificially introduced into cells.

Identifying the siRNA lengths that best
(60) suppressed gene expression in an in vitro *Drosophila* system was helpful in studies of invertebrate and plant systems, but methods for successfully using these extrinsic siRNAs in mammalian systems
(65) were elusive. Tuschl says that geneticists discovered the RNA silencing system, but "there was no biochemical system that showed [how] a specific long RNA is degraded" to siRNA. Brenda
(70) Bass, a Howard Hughes Medical Institute investigator at University of Utah, Salt Lake City, notes that "conventional methods of initiating RNAi with long double-stranded RNA do not work in
(75) most mammalian cells." The key to inhibition of mammalian gene expression was found in the shorter siRNA segments.

Nearly two years ago, Tuschl's team
(80) reported on the successful use of extrinsic siRNAs in a mammalian cell culture system. "Once we showed how it worked in flies ... we could go into mammalian cells and see if we...[could] silence a
(85) gene," says Tuschl. They could. "This paper provided the crucial information that allowed researchers to use RNA interference in mammalian cells," explains Bass, who wrote a commentary
(90) on the Nature paper. "This paper showed that ... an intermediate in the RNAi pathway (siRNA), could be successfully used to initiate RNAi in mammalian cells."

Reprinted with permission from *The Scientist,* January 13, 2003, Pages 36–37.

19. Tuschl said that this is the _____ paper "that is formal proof that siRNA can do gene silencing."

    (A) fourth

    (B) third

    (C) second

    (D) first

20. What is an siRNA?

    (A) Small initial RNA

    (B) Small inhibitory RNA

    (C) Sense inhibitory RNA

    (D) Sense initial RNA

21. Who first reported that double-stranded RNA could interfere with gene expression?

    (A) Fire and colleagues

    (B) Frist and colleagues

    (C) Free and colleagues

    (D) Frost and colleagues

22. What lysate system did Tuschl's group utilize in this study?

    (A) Drosophagia

    (B) Drisophagia

    (C) Drosophela

    (D) Drosophila

23. Which of the following did Tuschl and colleagues identify in this study?

    (A) Widths of siRNA

    (B) Lengths of siRNA

    (C) Lengths of mRNA

    (D) Lengths of tRNA

24. What is PTGS?

    (A) Posttranscriptional gene silencing

    (B) Posttranscriptional gene splicing

    (C) Posttranscriptional gene sensing

    (D) Posttranscriptional gene solutions

25. Where was the key to inhibition of mammalian gene expression found according to this passage?

    (A) Shorter iRNA segments

    (B) Shorter sRNA segments

    (C) Shorter siRNA segments

    (D) Shorter mRNA segments

26. What can cause direct gene silencing in mammalian cells without interference that kills the cells?

    (A) mRNA

    (B) siRNA

    (C) iRNA

    (D) siDNA

27. How many fragments of nucleoxide duplexes of sense and antisense RNA are necessary for the suppression of gene expression by RNA?

    (A) 20 or 22

    (B) 19 or 20

    (C) 21 or 23

    (D) 21 or 22

28. What type of cells was used in this study?

    (A) Fly and mammalian cells

    (B) Fly cells

    (C) Mammalian cells

    (D) Cell cultures

29. What type of cells did Tuschl's group first work with before progressing to mammalian cells?

    (A) Rats

    (B) Flies

    (C) Mice

    (D) Guinea pigs

30. What type of pathway did the Nature manuscript show could be successful in initiating RNAi in mammalian cells?

    (A) pRNA

    (B) tRNA

    (C) mRNA

    (D) siRNA

QUESTIONS 31–37 ARE BASED ON THE FOLLOWING PASSAGE.

Accelerating X-ray Crystallography

For years, the process of X-ray crystallography has moved at a tortoise's pace.
(5) "When I started in the field, it would typically take 20 person-years to produce a complete atomic model of one single protein. It was like a traffic jam in New York City. Every single part of the
(10) process was slow," says Stephen Burley, chief scientific officer and senior vice president of research at San Diego-based Structural GenomiX. The biggest holdup: obtaining a suitable crystal.

(15) Researchers can spend weeks or even months searching for optimal crystallization conditions. "You need a crystal and without a crystal you have nothing to do," explains Tom Hurley, professor
(20) of biochemistry and molecular biology at Indiana University. Other bottlenecks include data collection and data analysis.

Now the biotech industry and some
(25) academics are trying to kick the process up to hare speed. New high-throughput (HT) methods being developed will dramatically improve the pace at which researchers collect and analyze data on
(30) larger and more poorly diffracting proteins, macromolecular complexes, and nucleic acids. This improvement will transform the labor-intensive and time-consuming process of molecular struc-
(35) ture determination by X-ray crystallography into a powerful and viable method for advancing functional genomics, and ultimately, for translating raw genomic information into new pharmaceuticals.

(40) "The whole notion is to do more, faster, using automation as much as possible," explains Mark Rould, director of the University of Vermont's Center for X-ray Crystallography and assistant pro-
(45) fessor of molecular physiology and biophysics at the school's college of medicine. "Crystallography has gone from solving a structure once every decade to solving 75 percent of the projects in the
(50) lab within a week of collecting the data," explains Hurley.

SCHOLARLY DEBATE: Not everyone agrees about the feasibility and benefits of HT X-ray crystallography; some con-
(55) sider the goal of Structural GenomiX—5,000 proteins in five years—overly ambitious. Crystallographer Gongyi Zhang, National Jewish Medical and Research Center and University of Colo-
(60) rado Health Sciences Center, Denver, says that crystallization was, is, and will continue to be a rate-limiting step. Eventually, he says, biotech companies will fail to keep the pace they have been
(65) bragging about. Hurley, who believes HT techniques "will lead to a huge explosion of understanding in biochemistry," says that considerable development is still needed before leaping from struc-
(70) tural determination to drug design.

Reprinted from *The Scientist,* January 13, 2003, Page 39.

31. How many person-years did it take to produce a complete atomic model of a single protein?

    (A) Ten
    (B) Fifteen
    (C) Twenty
    (D) Twenty-five

32. According to this passage, what are two bottlenecks researchers must face when searching for optimal crystallization conditions?

    (A) Funds for research
    (B) Data collection
    (C) Data analysis
    (D) B and C

33. What does Gongyi Zhang say will continue to be a rate-limiting step?

    (A) Crystallization
    (B) Polymorphism
    (C) Cost of finding the best crystallization process
    (D) HT techniques

34. What does HT methods refer to?

    (A) High-temperature methods
    (B) High-throughput methods
    (C) Hard-throughput methods
    (D) High-theoretical methods

35. Crystallography has progressed from solving a structure once every decade to solving _____ of the projects.

    (A) 25 percent
    (B) 50 percent
    (C) 70 percent
    (D) 75 percent

36. According to Stephen Burley, chief scientific officer of Structural GenomiX, the biggest holdup is obtaining a suitable

    (A) crystal.
    (B) molecule.
    (C) atom.
    (D) ion.

37. The improvements in the process of molecular structure determination by X-ray crystallography will ultimately result in translation of

    (A) raw genomic information into new pharmaceuticals.
    (B) crystallization information into new pharmaceuticals.
    (C) raw genetic information into new pharmaceuticals.
    (D) raw information into new pharmaceuticals.

QUESTIONS 38–45 ARE BASED ON THE FOLLOWING PASSAGE.

Crystal Structure of Escherichia coli MscS, a Voltage-Modulated and Mechanosensitive Channel

(5) The mechanosensitive channel of small conductance, MscS, was identified by Kung and coworkers as a stretch-activated channel present in the inner membrane of *E. coli*. The MscS channel is characterized by a conductance of ~1 nS,

(10) with a slight preference for anions; this is substantially larger than the conductances of typical eukaryotic ion channels (1 to 30 pS), but smaller than the ~3 nS, nonselective conductance observed for

(15) the prokaryotic MscL (large conductance) mechanosensitive channel. Both MscS and MscL are intrinsically mechanosensitive, opening in response to stretching of the cell membrane with-

(20) out the requisite participation of cytoskeletal or other components. The pressure threshold for MscS opening is ~50 percent that of MscL, which in turn opens at pressures near the rupture point

(25) of the bilayer. The properties of these channels likely reflect their involvement in the cellular response to rapid decreases in external osmolarity, and the two channels share the ability to par-

(30) tially compensate for the deletion of the other. The gene encoding the MscS channel, yggB, was identified by Booth and coworkers; the *E. coli* protein, with 286 amino acids is predicted from hydr-

(35) opathy analyses to have three transmembrane helices and exhibits no detectable sequence similarities to the smaller (136 residues) MscL. In common with MscL and other prokaryotic chan-

(40) nels, such as KcsA, MscS exists as a homo-oligomer. However, MscS has a far greater distribution than MscL throughout eubacteria, and has also been identified in Archaea and at least some

(45) eukaryotes.

The conductances of gated channels such as MscS are regulated by conformational switching of the protein structure between open and closed states.

(50) This switching responds to changes in environmental conditions, including applied tension (mechanosensitive channels), variation in membrane potential (voltage-gated channels), and binding of

(55) ligands (ligand-gated channels). In recent years, progress has been made in defining the structural basis of channel gating. After the structure of the closed state of MscL was determined, detailed

(60) models were described for the structure of the open state and the coupling between membrane tension and structure. Structural aspects of the mechanism of ligand gating have been established for

(65) opening a prokaryotic potassium channel by proton binding to the channel and by calcium binding to an extramembrane domain. Although considerable insights into the mechanism of voltage-depen-

(70) dent gating have been achieved, to date, no structures of a voltage-gated system have been described.

Reprinted with permission from *Science,* Vol. 298, November 22, 2002, Page 1582, American Association for the Advancement of Science.

38. The conductances of gated channels such as _____ are regulated by conformational switching of the protein structure between open and closed states.

    (A) KcsA
    (B) MscS
    (C) MscL
    (D) mRNA

39. A mechanosensitive channel of small conductance is known as

    (A) MscL.
    (B) mRNA.
    (C) KcsA.
    (D) MscS.

40. MscS channel is characterized by a conductance of

    (A) ~ 1 nS.
    (B) ~ 2 nS.
    (C) ~ 3 nS.
    (D) ~ 4 nS.

41. Which of the following best describes the status of structures of a voltage-gated system?

    (A) Three structures have been described.
    (B) Two new structures have been described.
    (C) One new structure has been described.
    (D) No structures have been described.

42. Both MscS and MscL are _____ mechanosensitive.

    (A) extrinsically
    (B) intrinsically
    (C) extrinsically and intrinsically
    (D) None

43. Which of the following best describes the structural aspects of the mechanism of ligand gating established for opening a prokaryotic potassium channel by proton binding to the channel and by calcium binding to an extramembrane domain?

    (A) Protein binding to the channel
    (B) Peptide binding to the channel
    (C) Proton binding to the channel
    (D) Protase binding to the channel

44. According to this passage, how many amino acids does the *E. coli* have?

    (A) 236 amino acids
    (B) 286 amino acids
    (C) 256 amino acids
    (D) 268 amino acids

45. What is the pressure threshold for MscS compared to that of MscL?

    (A) ~ 20 percent of that of MscL
    (B) ~ 30 percent of that of MscL
    (C) ~ 40 percent of that of MscL
    (D) ~ 50 percent of that of MscL

QUESTIONS 46–48 ARE BASED ON THE FOLLOWING PASSAGE.

Much of the pharmacy profession has adopted the concept of pharmaceutical care to improve the outcome of drug therapy. Pharmaceutical care is defined
(5) as "the responsible provision of drug therapy for the purpose of achieving definite outcomes that improve a patient's quality of life." Using this model, pharmacists in numerous settings have
(10) sought to reduce drug-related morbidity and mortality.

Studies of pharmaceutical care, however, have been based on only one study site, did not have a control group, or did
(15) not randomize patient assignment. Another common problem with previous research is that interventions were not focused necessarily on patients who most likely would benefit from clinical phar-
(20) macy services. This study, which sought to overcome these limitations, is referred to as the IMPROVE study (Impact of Managed Pharmaceutical Care on Resource Utilization and Outcomes in Vet-
(25) erans Affairs Medical Centers). Its purpose was to determine if clinical pharmacists could affect economic resource use and humanistic outcomes in a population of veterans identified to be at high
(30) risk to experience a medication-related problem.

This was a prospective, multi-site, randomized controlled trial. Its background and study design are described else-
(35) where. Sites selected were Veterans Affairs medical centers (VAMCs) that were recruited for participation by completing an invitation and a site survey. A questionnaire was developed to capture
(40) data to characterize the scope of pharmaceutical services and was mailed to 714 centers.

46. Much of the pharmacy profession has adopted the concept of
  (A) quality of life.
  (B) pharmaceutical sciences.
  (C) pharmaceutical care.
  (D) economic outcomes.

47. Which of the following was a problem with studies of pharmaceutical care?
  (A) Did not have a control
  (B) Were not randomized
  (C) Were not randomized as to sites
  (D) Were focused on patients who would not benefit from pharmaceutical care

48. This _____ study sought to overcome the problems of previous studies.
  (A) EXCLUDE
  (B) INCLUDE
  (C) IMPROVE
  (D) EXPORT

BIOLOGY

58 Questions • 35 Minutes

> **Directions:** Choose the one best answer to each of the following questions.

1. Which of the following is NOT an example of an exocrine gland?

    (A) Merocrine

    (B) Halocrine

    (C) Endocrine

    (D) Apocrine

2. Which of the following is true regarding an animal cell membrane?

    (A) The interior is hydrophilic and the exterior is hydrophobic.

    (B) The interior is hydrophilic and the exterior is hydrophilic.

    (C) The interior is hydrophobic and the exterior is hydrophilic.

    (D) The interior is hydrophobic and the exterior is hydrophobic.

3. Which of the following is incorrect regarding membrane transport?

    (A) Simple diffusion involves movement of molecules from an area of high concentration to an area of lower concentration.

    (B) Facilitated diffusion is the ATP-dependent movement of molecules or ions against a concentration gradient.

    (C) Filtration is when water and solutes are forced (high to low concentration) through a membrane by hydrostatic pressure.

    (D) Osmosis is the diffusion of water molecules through a selectively permeable membrane.

4. Which of the following is incorrect regarding cutaneous sensation?

    (A) Meissner's corpuscles are responsible for light-touch detection.

    (B) Pacinian corpuscles are located in dermal papillae.

    (C) Pacinian corpuscles are responsible for pressure detection.

    (D) Meissner's corpuscles are found in areas such as fingertips, palms, soles, and eyelids.

5. Which of the following is a function of the hormone calcitonin?

    (A) It causes a deposition of bone matrix by inhibiting bone resorption and increasing osteoblast activity.

    (B) It increases blood Ca^{++} via stimulation of bone resorption.

    (C) It is secreted by the parathyroid gland.

    (D) It promotes Ca^{++} reabsorption in the kidney tubules.

6. Which of the following allows for bone growth until adulthood?

    (A) Bone shaft

    (B) Periosteum

    (C) Bone marrow

    (D) Epiphyseal growth plate

7. Which of the following is least involved with muscle contraction?

   (A) ATP

   (B) Calcium

   (C) Actin

   (D) Potassium

8. Which neurotransmitter is involved in muscle contraction?

   (A) Acetylcholine

   (B) Serotonin

   (C) Dopamine

   (D) GABA

9. Which of the following is true regarding cellular energetics?

   (A) Aerobic glycolysis results in alcohol and lactic acid fermentation.

   (B) Lactic acid buildup results in muscle soreness and fatigue.

   (C) Cellular respiration results in 46 ATP molecules being produced from a single glucose molecule.

   (D) Glycolysis is the anaerobic conversion of 6-carbon sugar (e.g., glucose) to two pyruvate molecules, resulting in the formation of ATP.

10. Regarding the structure and function of neurons, all of the following are true EXCEPT

    (A) dendrites are neuron extensions that carry impulses to the cell body.

    (B) axons are neuron extensions that carry impulses away from the cell body.

    (C) Schwann cells in the central nervous system produce myelin.

    (D) there is only one axon per neuron.

11. The distribution of ions across the cell membrane determines the resting membrane potential (RMP) of a neuron. Which of the following is incorrect regarding the RMP?

    (A) K^+ is high inside the cell.

    (B) Na^+ is high inside the cell.

    (C) Cl^- is high outside the cell.

    (D) The Na^+K^+–ATPase pump is responsible for maintaining the RMP.

12. Movement of impulses from one neuron to another is known as synaptic transmission. Which of the following best describes the synapse?

    (A) The actual electrical impulse

    (B) The junction between two neurons

    (C) The terminal process of the neuron

    (D) The hormone response for impulse transmission

13. Which of the following best describes the process by which continual stimulation of the postsynaptic membrane is prevented?

    (A) Neurotransmitters are either destroyed by specific enzymes in the synaptic cleft or undergo reuptake into the presynaptic cleft.

    (B) Neurotransmitters diffuse from the synaptic cleft.

    (C) Neurotransmitters undergo non-enzymatic breakdown.

    (D) Neurotransmitters are either destroyed by specific enzymes in the synaptic cleft or undergo reuptake into the postsynaptic cleft.

14. Which of the following is incorrect regarding sensory receptors?

    (A) Mechanoreceptors respond to changes in pressure.

    (B) Thermoreceptors are the only somatic sensory receptors that do not undergo sensory adaptation.

    (C) Photoreceptors respond to light.

    (D) Nociceptor stimulation gives rise to pain sensation.

15. Analgesics are commonly used to reduce pain and inflammation. Which of the following is NOT considered an analgesic?

    (A) Ibuprofen

    (B) Tylenol

    (C) Aspirin

    (D) Lipitor

16. Sensory information received by the five special senses (hearing, vision, equilibrium, taste, and smell) is relayed to the brain by specific cranial nerves (CNs). Which of the following sense : cranial nerve associations is incorrect?

    (A) Smell : CN I

    (B) Hearing : CN VIII

    (C) Sight : CN II

    (D) Taste : CN X

17. Hormones are blood-borne messengers of the endocrine system. Which of the following is NOT an endocrine gland?

    (A) Pituitary

    (B) Thymus

    (C) Sebaceous

    (D) Testes

18. The hypothalamus triggers hormone release from the anterior pituitary. Which of the following is secreted by the hypothalamus?

    (A) Adrenocorticotropin hormone

    (B) Anti-diuretic hormone

    (C) Oxytocin

    (D) Aldosterone

19. The pancreas functions as an exocrine and an endocrine gland. Which of the following best describes the endocrine gland function of the pancreas?

    (A) The endocrine glands of the pancreas are known as Peyer's Patches.

    (B) The endocrine glands of the pancreas are known as Islets of Langerhans.

    (C) Insulin produced by b-cells increases blood glucose levels.

    (D) Glucagon produced by a-cells decreases blood glucose levels.

20. Arteries carry blood from the heart, and veins carry blood to the heart. In general, which of the following is true regarding oxygen and carbon dioxide levels carried by blood vessels?

    (A) Arteries carry blood that is *high* in carbon dioxide and *low* in oxygen.

    (B) Veins carry blood that is *high* in oxygen and *low* in oxygen.

    (C) Arteries carry blood that is *high* in oxygen and *low* in carbon dioxide.

    (D) Veins carry blood that is *high* in oxygen and carbon monoxide.

21. Which of the following separates the right atrium and ventricle?

    (A) Aortic semilunar valve

    (B) Tricuspid valve

    (C) Pulmonary semilunar valve

    (D) Bicuspid valve

22. Which of the following is known as the "pacemaker" of the heart?

    (A) Atrioventricular node

    (B) Purkinje fibers

    (C) Sinoatrial node

    (D) Atrioventricular bundle

23. Which of the following is NOT one of the three waves comprising a single heartbeat?

    (A) T wave

    (B) QRS complex

    (C) Z wave

    (D) P wave

24. Which of the following is incorrect regarding mean arterial blood pressure (MABP)?

    (A) MABP is maximum during systole.

    (B) MABP is minimum during diastole.

    (C) Normal MABP is 120 mm Hg/80 mm Hg.

    (D) Cardiac output is the product of heart rate and MABP.

25. Which of the following is NOT a hormone responsible for increasing blood pressure?

    (A) Epinephrine

    (B) Antidiruetic hormone

    (C) Aldosterone

    (D) Histamine

26. Which is neither a primary nor a secondary organ of the lymphatic system?

    (A) Thymus

    (B) Lymph nodes

    (C) T-cells

    (D) Spleen

27. Which of the following is NOT a function of the lymphatic system?

    (A) Prevents edema by returning excess interstitial fluid to the cardiovascular system

    (B) Returns proteins that leak out of the blood vessel capillaries

    (C) Transports water-soluble vitamins from the gastrointestinal system to the bloodstream

    (D) Transports foreign particles to the lymph nodes

28. Which of the following is the site of T-cell maturation?

    (A) Lymph node

    (B) Thymus

    (C) Red bone marrow

    (D) Spleen

29. Which of the following is NOT a component of the body's nonspecific immune response?

    (A) Inflammation

    (B) Fever

    (C) Phagocytosis

    (D) Antibodies

30. Which of the following cell types are considered antigen-presenting cells that trigger the specific immune response?

    (A) Macrophage

    (B) T-cell

    (C) B-cell

    (D) Neutrophil

31. B-cells secrete antibodies, known as immunoglobulins, which provide antibody-mediated immunity. Which of the following immunoglobulin is involved in the allergic reaction?

    (A) IgA

    (B) IgE

    (C) IgM

    (D) IgG

32. Which of the following is a function of salivary amylase?

    (A) Converts polysaccharides to disaccharides
    (B) Contracts gastroesophageal sphincter
    (C) Breaks down fats and triglycerides
    (D) Causes release of pancreatic juice into the duodenum

33. Which of the following is NOT a function of the liver?

    (A) Inactivates toxins
    (B) Filters old blood cells
    (C) Produces and secretes bile
    (D) Stores and concentrates bile between meals

34. Which of the following is the site where a majority of nutrients are absorbed?

    (A) Stomach
    (B) Large intestine
    (C) Colon
    (D) Small intestine

35. Which of the following best describes tidal volume?

    (A) Maximum volume of air that a person can expire after maximal inspiration
    (B) Volume of air that can be forcibly expired after the resting tidal volume has been expired
    (C) Volume of air entering the lungs during a single inspiration
    (D) Volume of air that can be inspired over and above the resting tidal volume

36. Alveoli are microscopic air sacs found in the lung. Which of the following is incorrect regarding the alveoli?

    (A) Alveoli are comprised of Type I and II alveolar cells.
    (B) Type I alveolar cells secrete surfactant.
    (C) Surfactant acts to decrease surface tension, facilitating gas exchange.
    (D) Alveolar macrophages remove foreign particles from the air spaces.

37. In a mixture of gases, the pressure exerted by each gas is independent of the pressure exerted by others. This is known as

    (A) Boyle's Law.
    (B) Dalton's Law.
    (C) Beer's Law.
    (D) Logan's Law.

38. Oxygen is transported in the blood bound to which of the following proteins?

    (A) Hemoglobin
    (B) Albumin
    (C) Alpha–1 acid glycoprotein
    (D) Transcortin

39. CO_2 produced by cellular respiration is enzymatically converted to carbonic acid, which rapidly dissociates to bicarbonate ion. The reaction is reversed in the lungs and CO_2 is expelled. Which of the following enzymes is crucial to this process?

    (A) Monoamine oxidase
    (B) Dopamine decarboxylase
    (C) Carbonic anhydrase
    (D) 11-beta hydroxysteroid dehydrogenase

40. Which of the following is responsible for regulation of red blood cell formation (erythropoiesis)?

    (A) Aldosterone

    (B) Erythropoietin

    (C) Renin

    (D) Angiotensin

41. Which of the following is NOT involved in urine formation?

    (A) Filtration

    (B) Secretion

    (C) Reabsorption

    (D) Micturition

42. Which of the following is considered the functional unit of the kidney?

    (A) Cortex

    (B) Nephron

    (C) Medulla

    (D) Loop of Henle

43. Which of the following is incorrect regarding the kidney's role in maintaining total body water balance?

    (A) Sodium reabsorption is an active process.

    (B) Hormonal control of sodium reabsorption occurs mainly in the loop of Henle.

    (C) Potassium ions serve as the counter-ion for sodium reabsorption in tubular epithelial cells.

    (D) The majority of sodium and water reabsorption occurs in the proximal tubule.

44. Which of the following is incorrect regarding meiosis?

    (A) Meiosis is a type of cell division that results in the formation of gametes, with half the number of chromosomes as the parent cell.

    (B) Human sex cells are diploid.

    (C) Fertilization results in a diploid zygote.

    (D) The genetic information found in chromosomes is known as DNA.

45. Which of the following is NOT a hormone involved in the development of sex characteristics?

    (A) Estrogen

    (B) Testosterone

    (C) Follicular stimulating hormone

    (D) Angiotensin

46. A mutation is an error found in the genetic code. Which of the following is the most common type of genetic variation?

    (A) DNA insertion

    (B) DNA deletion

    (C) Single nucleotide polymorphism (SNP)

    (D) Tandem repeat

47. Alleles are alternate forms of the same gene. For autosomal genes, we inherit one allele from our mother and one from our father. Regarding inheritance, which of the following is incorrect?

    (A) Phenotype is the manifested or expressed trait.

    (B) Genotype determines phenotype.

    (C) Homozygous means that we have inherited identical alleles.

    (D) Homozygotes and heterozygotes always display a different phenotype.

48. Thousands of chemical reactions occur throughout the body. Which of the following is incorrect regarding chemical reaction rates?

    (A) Higher reactant concentrations result in a more rapid reaction rate.

    (B) Higher required activation energy results in a more rapid reaction rate.

    (C) Lower temperature results in a lower reaction rate.

    (D) The presence of a catalyst results in a faster reaction rate.

49. Enzymes can be thought of as protein catalysts. Which of the following is incorrect regarding enzymes?

    (A) An enzyme undergoes no net chemical change as a result of the reaction it catalyzes.

    (B) An enzyme increases the rate of a reaction; however, it will not cause a reaction to occur that would not have occurred in its absence.

    (C) An enzyme affects the rate at which equilibrium is achieved and can thereby change the final equilibrium.

    (D) An enzyme lowers the activation energy.

50. The paradigm of molecular biology is the flow of genetic information from DNA to RNA and then to protein. Which of the following is incorrect regarding this paradigm?

    (A) DNA is composed of adenine, cytosine, thymine, and guanine.

    (B) The ribosome is the site of protein synthesis.

    (C) Messenger RNA carries the appropriate amino acid to the ribosome during protein synthesis.

    (D) Transfer of information from the gene to messenger RNA is known as transcription.

51. The function of the lysosome is

    (A) to break down bacteria and dead cell debris from engulfed cells.

    (B) to sort the different types of proteins received from the granular endoplasmic reticulum into vesicles to be delivered to other parts of the cell.

    (C) to detoxify cellular wastes such as hydrogen peroxide.

    (D) the site of lipid synthesis and storage and release of calcium ions involved in controlling cellular activities.

52. Interphase of the cell cycle is defined as

    (A) the period during which cell growth and DNA synthesis occur.

    (B) the period between the end of one cell division and the appearance of the structural changes that indicate the beginning of the next division.

    (C) the period comprised of the G0 and S phases.

    (D) the period comprised of the G1, S, and G2 phases.

53. What represents the largest energy store in the body?

    (A) Lactic acid

    (B) Glycogen

    (C) Glucose

    (D) Fat

54. Which of the following vitamins is NOT required for bone growth, repair, and remodeling?

    (A) Vitamin K

    (B) Vitamin B12

    (C) Vitamin C

    (D) Vitamin D

55. Men and women lose bone at the same rate throughout life.

    (A) True

    (B) False

56. Sensory adaptation is the process by which a sensory receptor becomes less stimulated following continuous stimuli. Which of the following types of receptors do NOT undergo sensory adaptation?

    (A) Thermoreceptors

    (B) Chemoreceptors

    (C) Nocioreceptors

    (D) Both A and C

57. B-cell maturation to antibody secreting cells takes place in which organ?

    (A) Bone marrow

    (B) Thymus

    (C) Spleen

    (D) Lymph nodes

58. Which of the following is NOT a steroid secreted by the adrenal glands?

    (A) Norepinephrine

    (B) Cortisol

    (C) Aldosterone

    (D) Androgens

QUANTITATIVE ABILITY

58 Questions • 50 Minutes

Directions: Choose the one best answer to each of the following questions.

1. $\left[\dfrac{4}{8} \times \dfrac{6}{12}\right] + \dfrac{1}{4} =$
   - (A) $\dfrac{1}{2}$
   - (B) $\dfrac{11}{24}$
   - (C) $\dfrac{25}{100}$
   - (D) $\dfrac{5}{20}$

2. $0.25\,(5 + 3) + 4 =$
   - (A) 6
   - (B) 3
   - (C) 12
   - (D) 12.25

3. $\dfrac{(4+8)}{0.4} - 1 =$
   - (A) 30
   - (B) 3
   - (C) 11
   - (D) 29

4. $\dfrac{(15-3)}{(2+4)} \times 2.5 =$
   - (A) 4.25
   - (B) 5
   - (C) 6.25
   - (D) 2

5. $5^3 + 5 =$
   - (A) 20
   - (B) 125
   - (C) 650
   - (D) 130

6. $2^3 \times 2^2 =$
   - (A) 32
   - (B) 10
   - (C) 16
   - (D) 48

7. $X^2 \times Y^{-2} =$
   - (A) $(XY)^4$
   - (B) $(XY)^{-4}$
   - (C) $\dfrac{X^2}{Y^{\frac{1}{2}}}$
   - (D) $\dfrac{X^2}{Y^2}$

8. $\sqrt[3]{8} =$
   - (A) 24
   - (B) 512
   - (C) 3
   - (D) 2

9. $\sqrt{2} \times \sqrt{6} \times \sqrt{3} =$
   - (A) 24
   - (B) 12
   - (C) 6
   - (D) 3

10. $\log_5(25) =$
    - (A) 5
    - (B) 2
    - (C) 1
    - (D) 2.5

11. Which of the following is a prime number?
    (A) 9
    (B) 0.5
    (C) 2^3
    (D) 11

12. $13 - |-2| + |-6| =$
    (A) 17
    (B) 5
    (C) 1
    (D) 21

13. The expression $5 \times [25 \times 8 \times (3+4)] = (5 \times 25) \times 8 \times (3 + 4)$ is an example of the
    (A) associative law of addition.
    (B) commutative law of multiplication.
    (C) associative law of multiplication.
    (D) commutative law of addition.

14. Evaluate the formula: $\dfrac{12+[15x-7y+2]}{8}$ for $x = 2$ and $y = 8$.
    (A) -3
    (B) $-4\frac{1}{2}$
    (C) -11
    (D) $-1\frac{1}{2}$

15. Evaluate the formula: $\dfrac{KL^2}{C}$ for $K = 5$, $L = 10$, and $C = 2$.
    (A) 1,000
    (B) 250
    (C) 25
    (D) 50

16. The volume of a cylinder is obtained as the product of π, its height (h), and its radius (r) squared. The corresponding formula is:
    (A) $\pi r \left(r^2 + h^2\right)^{\frac{1}{2}}$
    (B) $\pi r^2 h$
    (C) $2\pi rh$
    (D) πrh^2

17. Solve the following equation for x: $4x - 3 = -6x + 17$.
    (A) 10
    (B) 7
    (C) 12
    (D) 2

18. Solve the following equation for y: $\dfrac{(2y+3)}{5} - 10 = \dfrac{(4-3y)}{2}$.
    (A) 114
    (B) 24
    (C) 6
    (D) 9

19. Solve the following equation for z: $z + 5 = 4(z + 2) - (2z + 1)$.
    (A) 7
    (B) -2
    (C) 3
    (D) 2

20. John is now three times as old as Harry. Four years ago, John was five times as old as Harry was then. How old is John now?
    (A) 6 years old
    (B) 12 years old
    (C) 16 years old
    (D) 24 years old

21. Doug drove at a certain fixed speed for 2 hours. He then drove 20 miles per hour faster for 4 hours. The total distance covered was 320 miles. What speed, in miles per hour, did Doug maintain in the first leg of the trip?
    (A) 20 mph.
    (B) 30 mph.
    (C) 40 mph.
    (D) 50 mph.

22. Solve for Y: $5Y^2 = 10Y$. One solution is
    (A) 2
    (B) 5
    (C) 10
    (D) –5

23. Solve for Z: $aZ - b = cZ + d$.
    (A) $\dfrac{(d+b)}{(a-c)}$
    (B) $\dfrac{ac}{db}$
    (C) $\dfrac{(a-c)}{(d+b)}$
    (D) $\dfrac{(a-b)}{(c+d)}$

24. Solve for A: $8A - 17 > -7 + 3A$.
    (A) > 5
    (B) < 2
    (C) > -3
    (D) > 2

25. Solve for B: $\dfrac{B}{6} - \dfrac{B}{4} \geq 1$.
    (A) ≥ 6
    (B) ≤ -12
    (C) ≥ 12
    (D) ≤ 6

26. Solve for C: $3C - 18 < 8C - 3$.
    (A) < 6
    (B) < 8
    (C) > -3
    (D) < 3

27. Solve for Y: $Y^2 + 7Y + 10 = 0$. One of the roots is
    (A) 5
    (B) –2
    (C) 7
    (D) –4

28. Solve for x: $x(x - 12) = 0$. One of the roots is
    (A) –12
    (B) 6
    (C) 12
    (D) –4

29. Solve for K: $K^2 + 36 = 5K^2$. One of the solutions is
    (A) –3
    (B) 6
    (C) 4
    (D) 12

30. Solve the simultaneous equations for C: $B + 2C = 12$ and $-B + 4C = 0$.
    (A) 3
    (B) –3
    (C) 6
    (D) 2

31. Solve the simultaneous equations for B: $2A + B = -7$ and $A - B = 1$.
    (A) –3
    (B) 7
    (C) –4
    (D) 6

32. If a patient is to take 2 tablets every morning and 1 tablet every evening, how many tablets will be required for a 14-day supply?
    (A) 28
    (B) 14
    (C) 36
    (D) 42

33. A formula for preparation of 200 ml of a lotion calls for 16 g of calamine. How much calamine would be required to make 50 ml of the lotion?
    (A) 32 g
    (B) 8 g
    (C) 4 g
    (D) 12 g

34. How many grams of coal tar should be added to 450 grams of zinc oxide paste to prepare an ointment containing 10% coal tar?

   (A) 50 g

   (B) 45 g

   (C) 90 g

   (D) 10 g

35. What is the median test score in the set of scores: 98, 62, 77, 96, 86, 93, and 72?

   (A) 83

   (B) 86

   (C) 90

   (D) 77

36. In triangle ABC, $AC = BC$. If the angle C is 30°, what is the angle A?

   (A) 75°

   (B) 45°

   (C) 60°

   (D) 30°

37. What is the length of the diagonal of a rectangle whose sides are 6 cm and 8 cm in length?

   (A) 6 cm

   (B) 8 cm

   (C) 10 cm

   (D) 12 cm

38. What is the area of a circle inscribed in a square whose sides are of length 8 inches?

   (A) 64 sq. in.

   (B) 50.2 sq. in.

   (C) 38.6 sq. in.

   (D) 24.2 sq. in.

39. Below, lines A and B are parallel. How many degrees is the angle α formed by lines B and C?

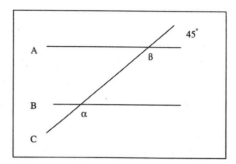

   (A) 45°

   (B) 150°

   (C) 90°

   (D) 135°

40. What is the area of a square inscribed in a circle of diameter 10?

   (A) 100

   (B) 50

   (C) 80

   (D) 200

41. The x- and y-coordinates of a point can be represented as (x, y). What is the distance between the two points $(-3, 2)$ and $(1, -1)$?

   (A) 5

   (B) 12

   (C) 7

   (D) 3.2

42. If the volume of a cube is 1,000 cubic inches, what is its surface area?

   (A) 100 sq. in.

   (B) 500 sq. in.

   (C) 600 sq. in.

   (D) 2,000 sq. in.

43. If a line is represented by the equation $Y = 5x + 25$, what is its x-intercept?

(A) 25

(B) −10

(C) −5

(D) 15

44. What is the equation for the straight line in the XY plot below?

XY Plot

(A) $Y = 2.5x + 25$

(B) $Y = 10x + 50$

(C) $Y = 25x − 10$

(D) $Y = 12.5x + 5$

QUESTION 45 IS BASED ON THE GRAPH BELOW.

Driving Speed

45. What is the slope of the straight line in the graph?

(A) 10

(B) 25

(C) 50

(D) 75

46. What is the diameter of the circle given by the equation $x^2 + y^2 − 36 = 0$?

(A) 36

(B) 18

(C) 12

(D) 6

47. Let f be a function defined by $f(x) = 2x^3 + 5x^2 + 15$. Find $f(6)$.

(A) 57

(B) 627

(C) 386

(D) 764

48. Find the value of: $\lim_{x \to 5} \dfrac{x^2 + 6}{x - 4}$.

(A) $+ \infty$

(B) 0

(C) 16

(D) 31

49. Find the derivative (i.e., $\frac{dy}{dx}$) of
$y = 6x^2 - 8x + 12$.
    (A) $12x - 8$
    (B) $6x - 8$
    (C) $3x^3 - 4x^2 + 12x$
    (D) 10

50. What is the value of the derivative of
$y = x^3 + 2x^2$ at $x = 5$?
    (A) 15
    (B) 225
    (C) 75
    (D) 95

51. Find the derivative of $y = (x^2 + 5)^3$.
    (A) $6x(x^2 + 5)^2$
    (B) $3(x^2 + 5)^2$
    (C) $2x$
    (D) $6x^2$

52. What is the derivative of $y = \sqrt{x-5}$?

    (A) $\sqrt{x-5}$

    (B) $\dfrac{1}{(2\sqrt{x-5})}$

    (C) $x\sqrt{x-5}$

    (D) $\dfrac{(x-5)^{\frac{3}{2}}}{2}$

53. Find $\frac{dy}{dx}$ for $y = \sin 2x + \cos^2 3x$.
    (A) $2(\cos 2x) - 6(\cos 3x)(\sin 3x)$
    (B) $\cos 2x + 2(\sin 3x)$
    (C) $2(\sin 2x) + 6(\cos 3x)$
    (D) $\tan 6x$

54. Find $\int 6x^2 dx$.
    (A) $12x + C$
    (B) $2x^3 + C$
    (C) $6x$
    (D) $3x$

55. Find $\int (4x^3 - 6x) dx$.
    (A) $12x^2 - 6 + C$
    (B) $x(4x^2 - 6)$
    (C) $x^4 - 3x^2 + C$
    (D) $24x + C$

56. Find $\int 3 \sin x \, dx$.
    (A) $-3 \cos x + C$

    (B) $\dfrac{3}{2} \sin^2 x + C$

    (C) $\cos 3x + C$

    (D) $\left(\dfrac{3}{2}\right) \cos^2 x + C$

57. Evaluate the definite integral: $\int_{2}^{8} 9x^2 dx$.
    (A) 504
    (B) 216
    (C) 512
    (D) 1512

58. Find the area under the curve given by
$y = x^2 - 2x + 5$ above the x axis, and
between $x = 0$ and $x = 1$.

    (A) $\dfrac{13}{3}$

    (B) $\dfrac{7}{2}$

    (C) 4

    (D) 8

CHEMISTRY

58 Questions • 35 Minutes

Directions: Choose the one best answer to each of the following questions.

1. The binding strength (concentration at IC50) of a potential drug to its receptor is usually expressed in nM. A concentration of 1 nM is equal to
   (A) 10^{-3}M
   (B) 10^{-6}M
   (C) 10^{-9}M
   (D) 10^{-12}M

2. How much sodium hydroxide (Na = 23, O = 16, H = 1) is needed to make a 500 ml of 0.3M solution of sodium hydroxide?
   (A) 20 g
   (B) 12 g
   (C) 9 g
   (D) 6 g

3. A student mixes a 500 ml of 1M sodium chloride solution with a 200 ml of 2M sodium chloride solution, then adds water to make the final volume 2,000 ml. The final concentration of sodium chloride is
   (A) 0.9M
   (B) 0.45M
   (C) 0.25M
   (D) 0.2M

4. Solution A has a pH = 9, and solution B has a pH = 5; therefore,
   (A) both A and B are acidic.
   (B) both A and B are basic.
   (C) A is basic and B is acidic.
   (D) A is acidic and B is basic.

5. With regard to significant figures, the correct result of 10.3 + 1.52 + 3.014 should be
   (A) 14.8
   (B) 14.83
   (C) 14.834
   (D) 15

6. Oxygen-17 has 8 protons and 9 neutrons. How many electrons does it have?
   (A) 16
   (B) 9
   (C) 17
   (D) 8

7. Which of the following statement about isotopes is false?
   (A) They have the same valence.
   (B) They have the same number of electrons.
   (C) They have the same mass.
   (D) They have the same chemical property.

8. Name the hydrocarbon $CH_3(CH_2)_5CH_3$.
   (A) Heptane
   (B) Pentane
   (C) Octane
   (D) Decane

9. Which of the following statements about ethylene is false?
   (A) Atoms in double bonds are not free to rotate.
   (B) The bond length between the carbons is shorter than in ethane.
   (C) The carbon has an *sp* hybrid orbital.
   (D) It is a symmetric molecule.

10. CH_3- group is called the
    (A) methyl group.
    (B) methylene group.
    (C) methane group.
    (D) methine group.

11. Which symbols can be used to assign the absolute configuration of a chiral molecule?
    (A) E and Z
    (B) Syn and anti
    (C) Cis and trans
    (D) R and S

12. With regard to hybrid orbitals, which statement is true about the oxygen in water and the nitrogen in ammonia?
    (A) Both have *sp*.
    (B) Both have sp^2.
    (C) Both have sp^3.
    (D) Water has sp^2 and ammonia has sp^3.

13. The percent composition by mass of a compound is important to verify the purity of a compound. What is the percentage composition by mass of hydrogen in H_2O_2 (H = 1, and O = 16)?
    (A) 2%
    (B) 5.9%
    (C) 6.2%
    (D) 50%

14. The correct name for HOCl is
    (A) hypochlorous acid.
    (B) chlorous acid.
    (C) chloric acid.
    (D) perchloric acid.

15. The balanced equation for $KClO_3 \Rightarrow KCl + O_2$ is
    (A) $KClO_3 \Rightarrow KCl + 3O_2$
    (B) $2KClO_3 \Rightarrow 2KCl + O_2$
    (C) $2KClO_3 \Rightarrow KCl + 3O_2$
    (D) $2KClO_3 \Rightarrow 2KCl + 3O_2$

16. Which compound is classified as a weak electrolyte in solution?
    (A) Sodium hydroxide
    (B) Acetic acid
    (C) Hydrochloric acid
    (D) Sodium carbonate

17. By definition of Brønsted theory, $H_2PO_4^-$ is a(n)
    (A) acid only.
    (B) base only.
    (C) acid and a base.
    (D) None of the above

18. In the reaction of $2Ca(s) + O_2(g) \rightarrow 2CaO(s)$, which statement is false?
    (A) The calcium atom loses electrons.
    (B) The oxygen atom loses electrons.
    (C) The entropy decreases in the reaction.
    (D) Calcium is a reducing agent.

19. At 1 atm and 0°C, 1 g of hydrogen gas occupies a volume of (atomic weight of H = 1)
    (A) 11.2 l
    (B) 22.4 l
    (C) 1 l
    (D) 760 l

20. Under the same temperature and pressure, which statement is true about the effusion rates of nitrogen and oxygen molecules in gas state (atomic weight: O = 16 and N = 14)?

    (A) Nitrogen is faster.

    (B) Oxygen is faster.

    (C) The rates are the same.

    (D) It cannot be determined.

21. The maximum number of electrons present in the principle level for which $n = 2$ is

    (A) 2

    (B) 4

    (C) 6

    (D) 8

22. The exclusion principle, which states that no two electrons in an atom can have the same four quantum numbers, is associated with

    (A) Heisenberg.

    (B) Pauli.

    (C) Bohr.

    (D) Planck.

23. Which simple molecule does NOT have a planar geometry?

    (A) Benzene

    (B) BF_3

    (C) NH_3

    (D) Ethylene

24. Which molecule does NOT have a pi bond?

    (A) Methanol

    (B) Formaldehyde

    (C) Acetone

    (D) Naphthalene

25. Which atoms are least likely to form hydrogen bonding?

    (A) Fluorine

    (B) Nitrogen

    (C) Oxygen

    (D) Carbon

26. Acetic acid is soluble in nonpolar solvent such as benzene, because acetic acid

    (A) is a nonpolar molecule.

    (B) is an aromatic compound.

    (C) can react with benzene.

    (D) molecules can form Dimmer's.

27. In the *homolysis* process, red blood cells are placed in a water solution in which the cells swell and eventually burst. This process is based on the phenomena of osmosis. The water solution in this process is considered to be a(n)

    (A) isotonic solution.

    (B) hypertonic solution.

    (C) hypotonic solution.

    (D) osmotic solution.

28. In reference to ion-product constant for water K_w, which statement is false?

    (A) $K_w = [H^+][OH^-]$.

    (B) K_w is temperature dependent.

    (C) K_w does not depend on pH.

    (D) K_w is pressure dependent.

29. At 25°C, the $[OH^-]$ concentration of a solution with pH = 4 is

    (A) 10^{-12}M

    (B) 10^{-10}M

    (C) 10^{-7}M

    (D) 10^{-4}M

30. Pick out the false statement about acid and base.

    (A) The stronger the acid, the stronger its conjugate base.

    (B) Strong acids are strong electrolytes.

    (C) NH_4^+ is the conjugate acid of NH_3.

    (D) H_3O^+ is the strongest acid that can exist in aqueous solution.

31. Oxides can be classified as acidic, basic, and amphoteric based on their reaction with water. Which of the following oxides is NOT an acidic oxide?

    (A) CO_2

    (B) As_2O_3

    (C) CaO

    (D) SO_2

32. For a 0.1M solution of weak acid HA, which is true?

    (A) pH = 1

    (B) pH > 1

    (C) pH < 1

    (D) It cannot be determined.

33. Considering $K_a = 4.9 \times 10^{-10}$ for HCN and $K_b = 1.8 \times 10^{-5}$ for NH_3, which statement about NH_4CN is true? (Hint: No calculation is necessary.)

    (A) The solution is basic.

    (B) The solution is acidic.

    (C) The solution is neutral.

    (D) It cannot be determined.

34. Which of the following solutions is NOT a buffer system?

    (A) CH_3COONa/CH_3COOH

    (B) $KClO_4/HClO_4$

    (C) KH_2PO_4/H_3PO_4

    (D) NH_3/NH_4NO_3

35. When 18 g of water vapor condense to 18 g of water, the entropy

    (A) equals to 1 mol.

    (B) does not change.

    (C) increases.

    (D) decreases.

36. Mercury (Hg) is the only metal that exists as a liquid at room temperature. The two oxidation states in which mercury exists are

    (A) divalent and tetravalent.

    (B) monovalent and divalent.

    (C) monovalent and trivalent.

    (D) divalent and trivalent.

37. With regard to halogens, which of the following statement is false?

    (A) Atomic radius increases as F < Cl < Br < I.

    (B) Acid strength of hydrogen halides increases as HF < HCl < HBr < HI.

    (C) All halogens form diatomic molecules in their elemental state.

    (D) All halogens can have oxidation number of +7 in their compounds.

38. All of the following are properties of hydrogen peroxide EXCEPT it

    (A) is a planar molecule in geometry.

    (B) can act as an oxidation agent.

    (C) can act as a reducing agent.

    (D) is easily miscible with water.

39. The decay of carbon isotope ^{14}C is used to determine the ages of certain objects. The ^{14}C isotope (atomic mass = 14, atomic number = 6) decays to ^{14}N (atomic mass = 14, atomic number = 7) with an emission of a particle. This particle is mostly likely a(n)

    (A) proton.

    (B) neutron.

    (C) electron.

    (D) α particle.

40. Which of the following statements about rotation around the chemical bond is false?

    (A) Atoms in double bonds are not free to rotate.

    (B) Atoms in a ring are not free to rotate.

    (C) Atoms in single bonds are free to rotate.

    (D) Atoms in triple bonds are free to rotate.

41. The number of structural isomers that C_5H_{12} can have is

    (A) 2

    (B) 3

    (C) 4

    (D) 5

42. The two geometric isomers of dibromoehtylene, BrHC = CHBr, are called

    (A) R- and s-isomers.

    (B) O- and p-isomers.

    (C) Cis- and trans-isomers.

    (D) N- and t-isomers.

43. What functional group does molecule $CH_2OHCOCH=CHCHO$ NOT have?

    (A) Ketone

    (B) Hydroxyl

    (C) Aldehyde

    (D) Ester

44. If H_2SO_4 is sulfuric acid, which of the following choices is sulfurous acid?

    (A) H_2SO_3

    (B) H_2S

    (C) H_3SO_3

    (D) H_3SO_4

45. In the reaction of $(CH_3)_2C=CH-CH_3 + HBr \rightarrow (CH_3)_2CBr–CH_2CH_3$, the hydrogen from HBr goes to the CH instead of C in the double bond. This is known as

    (A) Avogadro's law.

    (B) Markovnikov's rule.

    (C) Boyle's law.

    (D) Saytzeff's rule.

46. In which compound does the carbon have the highest positive oxidation number?

    (A) Carbon dioxide

    (B) Methanol

    (C) Formic acid

    (D) Methane

47. The esterification reaction converts alcohol to esters. For the reaction $CH_3COOH + CH_3CH_2OH \rightarrow CH_3COOCH_2CH_3 + H_2O$, which reactant(s) provide the –OH group?

    (A) CH_3CH_2OH

    (B) CH_3COOH

    (C) Half of CH_3CH_2OH and half of CH_3COOH

    (D) None of the above

48. In which order does the acidity increase for the following compounds?

    (A) Methanol < acetic acid < phenol

    (B) Acetic acid < methanol < phenol

    (C) Phenol < methanol < acetic acid

    (D) Methanol < phenol < acetic acid

49. The Tollen's test (silver-mirror test) will generally provide positive results for which group of compounds?

    (A) Esters

    (B) Amines

    (C) Ketones

    (D) Aldehyde

50. For a compound with three nonidentical asymmetric carbon atoms, the maximum number of possible stereoisomers is
    (A) 3
    (B) 6
    (C) 8
    (D) 9

51. Glucose is the key sugar of the body and known as the "blood sugar." Which is NOT a property of this compound?
    (A) It is optically active.
    (B) It is sweeter than sucrose.
    (C) It gives positive results for Tollen's test.
    (D) It can be reduced by H_2/Pt to a polyhydroxy alcohol.

52. Which amino acid is most likely to be classified as neutral amino acid?
    (A) Glycine
    (B) Lysine
    (C) Arginine
    (D) Histidine

53. Amides may have all of the following formulas EXCEPT
    (A) $R-CO-NH_2$
    (B) $R-CO-NHR$
    (C) $R-CO-NR_3$
    (D) $R-CO-NR_2$

54. How many isomers does trichlorobenzene have?
    (A) 2
    (B) 3
    (C) 4
    (D) 5

55. In organic chemistry, the Diels-Alder reaction involves a(n)
    (A) carboxylic acid and an alcohol.
    (B) alkene and a halogen.
    (C) acid and a base.
    (D) alkene and a diene.

56. Lipids are the major components of cell membranes. Which of the following compounds can NOT be classified as a lipid?
    (A) Fatty acids
    (B) Steroids
    (C) Starch
    (D) Cholesterol

57. A primary amine has at least 2 hydrogens attached to the nitrogen atom. A tertiary amine has
    (A) no hydrogen attached to the nitrogen atom.
    (B) only 1 hydrogen attached to the nitrogen atom.
    (C) 2 hydrogens attached to the nitrogen atom.
    (D) 3 hydrogens attached to the nitrogen atom.

58. In proteins, the α-helix and β-sheet refer to what level of protein structure?
    (A) Primary structure
    (B) Secondary structure
    (C) Tertiary structure
    (D) All of the above

VERBAL ABILITY

58 Questions • 35 Minutes

Directions: Choose the word that best completes the analogy.

1. LIBELOUS : CALUMNIOUS ::
   APPLAUDING :
   - (A) adulating
   - (B) invidious
   - (C) traducing
   - (D) detracting

2. MATRIARCH : DOWAGER ::
   DIVORCE :
   - (A) dame
   - (B) elope
   - (C) dowry
   - (D) sunder

3. PHYSICIAN : SAWBONES ::
   PHARMACIST :
   - (A) surgeon
   - (B) doc
   - (C) apothecary
   - (D) physic

4. PILASTER : COLUMN :: DOCK :
   - (A) pier
   - (B) pile
   - (C) boat
   - (D) piffle

5. ENCUMBERANCE : IMPEDANCE ::
   RESULT :
   - (A) assist
   - (B) assistance
   - (C) catalyst
   - (D) sequence

6. FERINE : BESTIAL :: FERTILE :
   - (A) fecund
   - (B) infertile
   - (C) sterile
   - (D) animal

7. CARBUNCLE : FURUNCLE ::
   AUBERGE :
   - (A) carburetor
   - (B) caravansary
   - (C) dimple
   - (D) doldrum

8. DEARTH : ABSENCE :: DEAN :
   - (A) leader
   - (B) follower
   - (C) professor
   - (D) actor

9. ENGROSS : DISPERSE :: ENGAGING :
   - (A) gross
   - (B) bewilder
   - (C) loathsome
   - (D) inscribe

10. FANCIER : AMATEUR ::
    WALLFLOWER :
    - (A) dancer
    - (B) imaginary
    - (C) enthusiast
    - (D) caprice

11. OYSTER : FORTE :: JOHN DORY :
    - **(A)** shrimp
    - **(B)** lobster
    - **(C)** crab
    - **(D)** fish

12. SLEIGHT : ADROITNESS :: MENIAL :
    - **(A)** dray horse
    - **(B)** pony
    - **(C)** mule
    - **(D)** bay

13. TREATISE : MONOGRAPH ::
    AGREEMENT :
    - **(A)** contract
    - **(B)** vows
    - **(C)** dissent
    - **(D)** telegraph

14. VORACIOUS : EDACIOUS ::
    VORTEX :
    - **(A)** bodacious
    - **(B)** maelstrom
    - **(C)** vulturous
    - **(D)** votary

15. WAGGERY : EARNEST :: WAGGLE :
    - **(A)** switch
    - **(B)** vulpine
    - **(C)** impishness
    - **(D)** ludicrous

16. LEXICON : WORDSTOCK :: LIAR :
    - **(A)** honest
    - **(B)** wordy
    - **(C)** wordsmith
    - **(D)** perjurer

17. TACIT : EXPLICIT :: TACKY :
    - **(A)** expressed
    - **(B)** implicit
    - **(C)** categorical
    - **(D)** modish

18. XANTHIPPE : SHREW ::
    WRECKAGE :
    - **(A)** sabotage
    - **(B)** shred
    - **(C)** screen
    - **(D)** sardonic

19. ZANY : HARLEQUIN :: THESPIAN :
    - **(A)** buffoon
    - **(B)** mummer
    - **(C)** drummer
    - **(D)** theatric

20. UTTERANCE : SILENCE ::
    ANNIHILATE :
    - **(A)** abolish
    - **(B)** extirpate
    - **(C)** invent
    - **(D)** salient

21. SLOTH : SEDULITY :: HARE :
    - **(A)** assiduity
    - **(B)** assiduousness
    - **(C)** diligence
    - **(D)** slowpoke

22. RUMINATE : MEDIATE ::
    RECREANT :
    - **(A)** perfidious
    - **(B)** recreate
    - **(C)** revolve
    - **(D)** revolt

23. POLITIC : EXPEDIENT :: POLITY :
    - **(A)** course
    - **(B)** tact
    - **(C)** polar
    - **(D)** civil

24. IRKSOME : ENGROSSING :: IRASCIBLE :
    (A) exciting
    (B) tolerant
    (C) hateful
    (D) tiresome

25. HONED : KEEN :: HORRID :
    (A) lurid
    (B) lean
    (C) mean
    (D) hewn

26. BALMY : MILD :: FAITHFUL :
    (A) explosive
    (B) docile
    (C) talkative
    (D) staunch

27. HOPE : PLEASURE :: DESPONDENCY :
    (A) frolic
    (B) gratification
    (C) joy
    (D) anguish

28. SCEPTER : AUTHORITY :: SCALES :
    (A) weight
    (B) justice
    (C) commerce
    (D) greed

29. ARCHIPELAGO : ISLAND :: GALAXY :
    (A) universe
    (B) space
    (C) star
    (D) Milky Way

30. FEAST : MEAL :: VELLUM :
    (A) paper
    (B) fur
    (C) cotton
    (D) forest

31. LEAP : STRIDE :: JUMP :
    (A) fall
    (B) step
    (C) skip
    (D) bound

32. LAMP : LIGHT :: CHAIR :
    (A) ottoman
    (B) table
    (C) back
    (D) seat

33. ABUNDANCE : ABROGATE :: DEARTH :
    (A) deny
    (B) establish
    (C) abstain
    (D) absolve

34. POUND : KILOGRAM :: WEIGHT :
    (A) mass
    (B) area
    (C) volume
    (D) capacity

35. INNING : BASEBALL :: ERA :
    (A) time
    (B) midnight
    (C) history
    (D) chronology

36. EVIL : EXORCISE :: BREAD :
    (A) carbohydrate
    (B) break
    (C) sandwich
    (D) shred

37. WIND : DEFICIT :: EROSION :
    (A) spending
    (B) appreciation
    (C) borrowing
    (D) employment

38. RAISIN : GRAPE :: PRUNE :
    (A) apricot
    (B) currant
    (C) plum
    (D) berry

39. SAFE : NECKLACE ::
    COMBINATION :
    (A) torque
    (B) bangle
    (C) circlet
    (D) clasp

40. BINDING : BOOK :: WELDING :
    (A) box
    (B) tank
    (C) chair
    (D) wire

41. EMINENT : LOWLY :: FREQUENT :
    (A) often
    (B) frivolous
    (C) rare
    (D) soon

FOR QUESTIONS 42–58, CHOOSE THE WORD OR SET OF WORDS THAT BEST COMPLETES THE SENTENCE.

42. Although _____ continues on minor points, the _____ themes of the General's plan have been accepted.
    (A) discussion .. peripheral
    (B) debate .. central
    (C) dissention .. cultural
    (D) agreement .. basic

43. Recent advances in research methodologies have created excitement in academic circles and have _____ greater interest in funding new research projects in the field.
    (A) stymied
    (B) intensified
    (C) magnified
    (D) engendered

44. Although the boom appeared to still be in full swing, in the latter years of the decade, most economic indicators pointed to _____ times ahead.
    (A) leaner
    (B) profitable
    (C) healthy
    (D) aberrant

45. Though often crude and overly _____, early theories of biogenesis were important for the _____ of the question of life's origin.
    (A) dramatic .. institutionalization
    (B) hypothetical .. clarification
    (C) inscrutable .. illumination
    (D) simplistic .. advancement

46. The lawyer's argumentation was _____ and factually misleading, but these problems in his closing argument were masked by his _____ and superior mastery of the language.

(A) spurious .. elusiveness

(B) debonair .. equivocations

(C) duplicitous .. dissembling

(D) specious .. eloquence

47. The professor became _____ after attempting to explain the important concept multiple different ways, but her visible frustration only made the student less likely to _____ the material.

(A) belligerent .. understand

(B) stupefied .. comprehend

(C) vexed .. grasp

(D) agitated .. eschew

48. Mr. Thomas had, in his local community, earned the reputation as being somewhat of a miser, but a review of his financial records revealed he was actually a _____.

(A) maverick

(B) hooligan

(C) maestro

(D) spendthrift

49. Recent demographic shifts in the population of Country X have resulted in many traditional political alliances becoming _____ as nascent political parties _____ large swathes of the electoral landscape.

(A) obsolete .. secure

(B) dislodged .. provide

(C) unhinged .. procure

(D) solvent .. release

50. Many see the attempt to sway public _____, though ostensibly a process of popular persuasion, to be _____ since it has been undertaken employing questionable pretenses.

(A) consent .. disreputable

(B) opinion .. undemocratic

(C) disfavor .. impractical

(D) ill-will .. treacherous

51. The _____ feuds between rival factions of the company's board destroyed the effectiveness of the company's leadership.

(A) fatalistic

(B) infernal

(C) hegemonic

(D) internecine

52. Unlike his most recent predecessor, the newly elected mayor did not appoint friends and associates to high posts in the city government, but eschewed such _____ in favor of a _____-based appointment criteria.

(A) nepotism .. value

(B) cronyism .. merit

(C) favoritism .. work

(D) recidivism .. experience

53. Though customarily marked by deliberate and _____ prose, the author's most recent correspondence was convoluted and _____.

(A) terse .. tiresome

(B) genuine .. superfluous

(C) acidic .. prosaic

(D) succinct .. prolix

54. The demolition crew did not successfully _____ the building since two walls remained intact.

    (A) raze

    (B) construct

    (C) erect

    (D) incapacitate

55. The ethicist argued that the person in question was not _____ for the man's injury since it was an accident.

    (A) culpable

    (B) attributable

    (C) capable

    (D) actionable

56. The publicity surrounding the mismanagement of the company's capital _____ the company's credibility with investors, but the company remained solvent largely on account of its _____ market share.

    (A) belabored .. steady

    (B) aided .. climbing

    (C) lessened .. volatile

    (D) damaged .. stable

57. Though the official had hoped his speech would calm the citizenry, his assurances did not _____ the crowd's fears concerning the likelihood of the natural disaster recurring.

    (A) alter

    (B) assuage

    (C) increase

    (D) bolster

58. It is a commonly noted behavior for a younger sibling to _____ the behavior of an older sibling, taking on their mannerisms or sense of style.

    (A) antagonize

    (B) ridicule

    (C) improve

    (D) emulate

CRITICAL THINKING ESSAY

Time—30 Minutes

Directions: In this section, you will have 30 minutes to analyze and explain your views on one of the topics presented below. Read the statement carefully. Write only on the topic given.

Argumentative Topic:

The U.S. health-care system is strong. Defend this statement.

Problem-Solving Topic:

The U.S. health-care system could benefit from the changes outlined below.

ANSWER KEY AND EXPLANATIONS

Reading Comprehension

1.	B	11.	B	21.	A	31.	C	41.	D
2.	C	12.	B	22.	D	32.	D	42.	B
3.	D	13.	C	23.	B	33.	A	43.	C
4.	A	14.	B	24.	A	34.	B	44.	B
5.	C	15.	C	25.	C	35.	D	45.	D
6.	B	16.	B	26.	B	36.	A	46.	C
7.	A	17.	D	27.	D	37.	A	47.	A
8.	D	18.	C	28.	A	38.	B	48.	C
9.	C	19.	D	29.	B	39.	D		
10.	B	20.	B	30.	D	40.	A		

1. **The correct answer is (B).** The answer to the question is found in lines 63–66 of the paragraph: "Three problems lead to esophageal dysphagia: impaired esophageal peristaltic motility, esophageal obstruction, and acid reflux . . . ."

2. **The correct answer is (C).** The answer to the question is found in lines 25 and 26 of the paragraph: "The average esophagus is about 9 to 10 inches long . . . ."

3. **The correct answer is (D).** The answer to the question is found in line 4 of the paragraph: "Fifty pairs of muscles . . . ."

4. **The correct answer is (A).** The answer to the question is found in lines 17 and 18 of the paragraph: ". . . the pharynx, the canal that connects the mouth to the . . . ."

5. **The correct answer is (C).** The answer to the question is found in lines 44–47 of the paragraph: "The vast majority of disorders occur in the involuntary state 2 (oropharyngeal dysphagia) and stage 3 . . . ."

6. **The correct answer is (B).** The answer to the question is found in lines 59–61 of the paragraph: "Oropharyngeal dysphagia is the most common subtype observed among the elderly, ..."

7. **The correct answer is (A).** The answer to the question is found in lines 28 and 29 of the paragraph: ". . . through the upper esophageal sphincter, a one-way valve . . . ."

8. **The correct answer is (D).** The answer to the question is found in lines 20 and 21 of the paragraph: "The larynx, meanwhile, closes tightly . . . ."

9. **The correct answer is (C).** The answer to the question is found in lines 39 and 40 of the paragraph: "Injectable botulinum toxin type B solution (Myobloc, ..."

10. **The correct answer is (B).** The answer to the question is found in lines 16–19 of the paragraph: "Botulinum toxin type B, a neurotoxin produced by Clostridium botulinum, acts by blocking acetylcholine release at the neuromuscular junction."

11. **The correct answer is (B).** The answer to the question is found in lines 19–22 of the paragraph: "Botulinum toxin type B, unlike botulinum toxin type A, is available as a sterile solution for injection . . . ."

12. **The correct answer is (B).** The answer to the question is found in lines 4 and 5 of the paragraph: "Headache is the most common patient complaint reported . . . ."

13. **The correct answer is (C).** The answer to the question is found in lines 24–28 of the paragraph: "Because of differences in vehicles, dilution schemes, and laboratory protocols for determining the median lethal dose in mice, units of biological activity of botulinum toxin type B cannot be . . . ."

14. **The correct answer is (B).** The answer to the question is found in lines 47–50 of the paragraph: "The severity of headaches was recorded by the patient on a scale from 0–5, where 0 = no headache and 5 = severe headache. . . ."

15. **The correct answer is (C).** The answer to the question is found in lines 8–11 of the paragraph: ". . . whether primary headaches (such as tension headache, migraine headache, cluster headache, and rebound headache . . . ."

16. **The correct answer is (B).** The answer to the question is found in lines 51 and 52 of the paragraph: "Botulinum toxin type B was given every three . . . ."

17. **The correct answer is (D).** The answer to the question is found in lines 30–33 of the paragraph: "However, botulinum toxin type B 5,000 units/ml is generally considered to have a therapeutic effect . . . ."

18. **The correct answer is (C).** The answer to the question is found in line 41 of the paragraph: ". . . was used at a neurology clinic . . . ."

19. **The correct answer is (D).** The answer to the question is found in line 29 of the paragraph: "The first paper, Tuschl explains, 'is the . . . .'"

20. **The correct answer is (B).** The answer to the question is found in lines 23 and 24 of the paragraph: ". . . engineered small inhibitory RNAs (siRNAs) . . . ."

21. **The correct answer is (A).** The answer to the question is found in lines 6 and 7 of the paragraph: "After Fire and colleagues first reported . . . ."

22. **The correct answer is (D).** The answer to the question is found in lines 48 and 49 of the paragraph: "But Tuschl's group, using a *Drosopbila* lysate system . . . ."

23. **The correct answer is (B).** The answer to the question is found in line 59 of the paragraph: "Identifying the siRNA lengths that best . . . ."

24. **The correct answer is (A).** The answer to the question is found in lines 36 and 37 of the paragraph: ". . . occurring system, posttranscriptional gene silencing (PTGS) . . . ."

25. **The correct answer is (C).** The answer to the question is found in lines 75 and 76 of the paragraph: "The key to inhibition of mammalian gene . . . ."

26. **The correct answer is (B).** The answer to the question is found in line 32 of the paragraph: ". . . shows that siRNAs can direct gene . . . ."

27. **The correct answer is (D).** The answer to the question is found in lines 52 and 53 of the paragraph: ". . . . occurs when the RNA fragments are 21- or 22-nucleotide duplexes of sense and antisense RNA."

28. **The correct answer is (A).** The answer to the question is found in lines 82–84 of the paragraph: "'Once we showed how it worked in flies . . . we could go into mammalian cells and see if we. . . ."

29. **The correct answer is (B).** The answer to the question is found in lines 82 and 83 of the paragraph: "Once we showed how it worked in flies . . . ."

30. **The correct answer is (D).** The answer to the question is found in lines 85–93 of the paragraph: "This paper showed that . . . an intermediate in the RNAi pathway (siRNA), could be successfully used to initiate . . . ."

31. **The correct answer is (C).** The answer to the question is found in lines 5–7 of the paragraph: ". . . would typically take 20 person-years to produce. . . ."

32. **The correct answer is (D).** The answer to the question is found in lines 20–22 of the paragraph: "Other bottlenecks include data collection and data analysis."

33. **The correct answer is (A).** The answer to the question is found in lines 61 and 62 of the paragraph: ". . . says that crystallization was, is, and will continue to be a rate-limiting step."

34. **The correct answer is (B).** The answer to the question is found in lines 26 and 27 of the paragraph: ". . . high-throughput (HT) methods . . . ."

35. **The correct answer is (D).** The answer to the question is found in lines 48 and 49 of the paragraph: ". . . structure once every decade to solving 75 percent . . . ."

36. **The correct answer is (A).** The answer to the question is found in line 14 of the paragraph: ". . . obtaining a suitable crystal."

37. **The correct answer is (A).** The answer to the question is found in lines 37–39 of the paragraph: ". . . and ultimately, for translating raw genomic information into new pharmaceuticals."

38. **The correct answer is (B).** The answer to the question is found in lines 46 and 47 of the paragraph: "The conductances of gated channels such as MscS . . . ."

39. **The correct answer is (D).** The answer to the question is found in lines 4 and 5 of the paragraph: "The mechanosensitive channel of small conductance, MscS, was . . . ."

40. **The correct answer is (A).** The answer to the question is found in lines 9 and 10 of the paragraph: ". . . conductance of ~1 nS, with a slight preference for anions . . . ."

41. **The correct answer is (D).** The answer to the question is found in lines 70 and 71 of the paragraph: ". . . to date, no structure of a voltage-gated system . . . ."

42. **The correct answer is (B).** The answer to the question is found in lines 16–18 of the paragraph: "Both MscS and MscL are intrinsically mechanosensitive, ..."

43. **The correct answer is (C).** The answer to the question is found in lines 65–68 of the paragraph: ". . . a prokaryotic potassium channel by proton binding to the channel and by calcium binding to an extramembrane domain."

44. **The correct answer is (B).** The answer to the question is found in lines 33 and 34 of the paragraph: ". . . the *E. coli* protein, with 286 amino acids is predicted . . . ."

45. **The correct answer is (D).** The answer to the question is found in lines 22 and 23 of the paragraph: ". . . threshold for MscS opening is ~50 percent that of MscL, ..."

46. **The correct answer is (C).** The answer to the question is found in lines 1–4 of the paragraph: "Much of the pharmacy profession has adopted the concept of pharmaceutical care to improve the outcome of drug therapy."

47. **The correct answer is (A).** The answer to the question is found in lines 12–15 of the paragraph: "Studies of pharmaceutical care, however, have been based on only one study site, did not have a control group, or did not randomize patient assignment."

48. **The correct answer is (C).** The answer to the question is found in lines 20–25 of the paragraph: "This study, which sought to overcome these limitations, is referred to as the IMPROVE study (Impact of Managed Pharmaceutical Care on Resource Utilization and Outcomes in Veterans Affairs Medical Centers)."

answers

Biology

1.	C	13.	A	25.	D	37.	B	49.	B
2.	A	14.	B	26.	C	38.	A	50.	C
3.	B	15.	D	27.	C	39.	C	51.	A
4.	B	16.	D	28.	B	40.	B	52.	D
5.	A	17.	C	29.	D	41.	D	53.	D
6.	D	18.	A	30.	A	42.	B	54.	A
7.	D	19.	B	31.	B	43.	B	55.	B
8.	A	20.	C	32.	A	44.	B	56.	C
9.	A	21.	B	33.	D	45.	D	57.	C
10.	C	22.	C	34.	D	46.	C	58.	A
11.	B	23.	C	35.	C	47.	D		
12.	B	24.	D	36.	B	48.	B		

1. **The correct answer is (C).** Exocrine glands include merocrine, halocrine, and apocrine glands.

2. **The correct answer is (A).** According to the Fluid Mosaic Model, the cell membrane consists of a bilayer of phospholipid molecules with the *inner* membrane being hydrophilic and the *exterior* surface being hydrophobic.

3. **The correct answer is (B).** Facilitated diffusion is similar to simple diffusion except that carrier proteins are required for transport of molecules.

4. **The correct answer is (B).** *Pacinian* corpuscles are located in deep dermis and subcutaneous regions. *Meissner's* corpuscles are located in dermal papillae.

5. **The correct answer is (A).** Stimulation of Ca^{++} resorption in the kidney tubules is a function of the parathyroid hormone, which is secreted by the parathyroid gland.

6. **The correct answer is (D).** The *epiphyseal growth plate* is the portion of the epiphyses where active proliferation of cartilage takes place.

7. **The correct answer is (D).** Muscle contraction involves the interaction between actin and myosin. This interaction is facilitated by the presence of calcium and ATP.

8. **The correct answer is (A).** Acetylcholine (ACh) is released from a motor end fiber, causing stimulation of the sarcolemma of muscle fiber.

9. **The correct answer is (A).** *Glycolysis* is the aerobic conversion of a 6-carbon sugar (e.g., glucose) to two pyruvate molecules resulting in the formation of 38 ATP molecules from a single glucose molecule. *Anaerobic glycolysis* results in alcohol and lactic acid fermentation.

10. **The correct answer is (C).** *Myelin* is produced by oligodendrocytes in the central nervous system and Schwann cells in the peripheral nervous system.

11. **The correct answer is (B).** Na^+ is in high concentration outside the cell.

12. **The correct answer is (B).** The synapse is a specialized junction between two neurons where the impulse is transferred from the presynaptic neuron to the postsynaptic neuron.

13. **The correct answer is (A).** Neurotransmitter clearance from the synaptic cleft can occur via degradation by specific enzymes (e.g., acetylcholine is destroyed by

acetylcholinesterase) or reuptake into storage vesicles within the presynaptic membrane.

14. **The correct answer is (B).** Nociceptors do not undergo sensory adaptation, which is a phenomenon where stimulus response diminishes with constant stimulation.

15. **The correct answer is (D).** *Lipitor* is commonly used to lower cholesterol.

16. **The correct answer is (D).** Sense of taste is relayed via two pathways. The anterior $\frac{2}{3}$ of the tongue is associated with CN VII and the posterior $\frac{1}{3}$ of the tongue is associated with CN IX.

17. **The correct answer is (C).** *Sebaceous* glands are exocrine glands that secrete oil.

18. **The correct answer is (A).** *Anti–diruetic hormone* and *oxytocin* are secreted by the posterior pituitary gland. *Aldosterone* is secreted by the adrenal glands.

19. **The correct answer is (B).** The Islets of Langerhans are the endocrine glands of the pancreas. Insulin produced by the b-cells within the Islets of Langerhans functions to *decrease* blood glucose levels. Glucagon produced by the a-cells within the Islets of Langerhans functions to *increase* blood glucose levels.

20. **The correct answer is (C).** In general, arteries carry blood rich in oxygen and low in carbon dioxide. The reverse is true for veins.

21. **The correct answer is (B).** The pulmonary and aortic semilunar valves lie within the pulmonary trunk and the aorta, respectively. The bicuspid valve separates the left atrium and ventricle.

22. **The correct answer is (C).** The *atrioventricular node* serves as a delay signal that allows for ventricular filling. *Purkinje fibers* conduct the impulse into

the mass of ventricular muscle tissue. The *atrioventricular bundle* serves as an electrical connection between the atria and ventricles.

23. **The correct answer is (C).** The *T wave* represents ventricular repolarization. The *QRS complex* represents the onset of ventricular depolarization. The *P wave* represents atrial depolarization.

24. **The correct answer is (D).** Cardiac output is the product of heart rate and stroke volume.

25. **The correct answer is (D).** *Histamine* acts to decrease blood pressure.

26. **The correct answer is (C).** *T-cells* are specialized leukocytes that are involved in mediating the specific immune response.

27. **The correct answer is (C).** The *lymphatic system* is involved in transporting lipids and lipid-soluble vitamins absorbed in the gastrointestinal tract to the blood stream.

28. **The correct answer is (B).** T-cells undergo selection and maturation in the *thymus*.

29. **The correct answer is (D).** Antibodies are produced by β-cells and serve as an integral component of the specific immune response.

30. **The correct answer is (A).** The *macrophage* engulfs the foreign particle and presents surface antigen that is recognized by T-cells. β-cells respond to activated T-cells by secreting antibodies.

31. **The correct answer is (B).** *IgA* molecules help defend against bacterial cells and viruses. *IgM* molecules are the first to be secreted after antigen exposure. *IgG* molecules defend against bacterial cells, viruses, and toxins.

32. **The correct answer is (A).** *Gastrin* is responsible for gastroesophageal sphinc-

ter contraction. *Lipases* found in pancreatic juice are responsible for the breakdown of fats and triglycerides. *Secretin* stimulates the release of pancreatic juice into the duodenum.

33. **The correct answer is (D).** The *gallbladder* is responsible for bile storage and concentration between meals.

34. **The correct answer is (D).** The majority of nutrient absorption takes place in the *small intestine.*

35. **The correct answer is (C).** *Vital capacity* is the maximum volume of air that a person can expire after maximal inspiration. *Inspiratory reserve volume* is the volume of air that can be inspired over and above the resting tidal volume. *Expiratory reserve volume* is the volume of air that can be forcibly expired after the resting tidal volume has been expired.

36. **The correct answer is (B).** *Surfactant* is secreted by Type II alveolar cells.

37. **The correct answer is (B).** In a mixture of gases, the pressure exerted by any one gas is known as *partial pressure* (Dalton's Law). The partial pressures of oxygen and carbon dioxide determine the direction that a gas moves through a respiratory membrane.

38. **The correct answer is (A).** Oxygen is weakly bound to hemoglobin to form oxyhemoglobin.

39. **The correct answer is (C).** Overall reaction: $CO_2 + H_2O \leftrightarrow H_2CO_3 \leftrightarrow H^+ + HCO_3^-$. Carbonic anhydrase present in erythrocytes catalyzes the rate-limiting first reaction.

40. **The correct answer is (B).** Erthropoietin is a hormonal substance that is formed especially in the kidney and stimulates red blood cell formation.

41. **The correct answer is (D).** *Micturition* is the process of expelling urine from the bladder.

42. **The correct answer is (B).** The kidney contains approximately 1 million functional units called nephrons.

43. **The correct answer is (B).** Hormonal control of sodium reabsorption occurs mainly in the collecting ducts.

44. **The correct answer is (B).** Human sex cells (sperm and egg) are haploid. Haploid cells contain half the full complement of chromosomes (i.e., 23 chromosomes).

45. **The correct answer is (D).** *Angiotensin* is involved in sodium reabsorption by the kidney.

46. **The correct answer is (C).** SNPs represent the most common form of genetic variant and are estimated to occur approximately every 1,000 base pairs.

47. **The correct answer is (D).** *Homozygotes* and *heterozygotes* may display the same phenotype. For example, in the case of the presence of a dominant allele, an individual carrying the dominant allele (either homozygote or heterozygote) will display the same phenotype.

48. **The correct answer is (B).** The higher the required activation energy, the lower the reaction rate.

49. **The correct answer is (B).** An enzyme affects the rate at which equilibrium is achieved. However, it cannot change the final equilibrium.

50. **The correct answer is (C).** Transfer RNA carries the appropriate amino acid to the ribosome during protein synthesis.

51. **The correct answer is (A).** The Golgi apparatus is responsible for sorting different types of proteins received from the granular endoplasmic reticulum. Peroxisomes are responsible for detoxification of cellular wastes. Lipid synthesis and storage/release of calcium occurs in the agranular endoplasmic reticulum.

52. **The correct answer is (D).** Interphase is comprised of the G1, S, and G2 phases.

53. **The correct answer is (D).** Lactic acid is a waste product generated during anaerobic glycolysis. Glycogen represents a storage form of glucose. Glucose is the available source of energy.

54. **The correct answer is (A).** Vitamin K is used in the body to control blood clotting and is essential for synthesizing the liver protein that controls the clotting.

55. **The correct answer is (B).** Women lose bone more rapidly than men following menopause. However, bone loss is similar in men and women after the age of 70.

56. **The correct answer is (C).** Nocioreceptors respond to extreme (harmful) stimuli by producing the sensation of pain and do not undergo sensory adaptation.

57. **The correct answer is (C).** T-cell maturation and selection takes place in the thymus. The red bone marrow serves as a production site for B- and T-cells. Macrophages found in lymph nodes phagocytize foreign particles.

58. **The correct answer is (A).** Norepinephrine is a neurotransmitter involved in smooth muscle contraction.

Quantitative Ability

1.	A	13.	C	25.	B	37.	C	49.	A
2.	A	14.	D	26.	C	38.	B	50.	D
3.	D	15.	B	27.	B	39.	D	51.	A
4.	B	16.	B	28.	C	40.	B	52.	B
5.	D	17.	D	29.	A	41.	A	53.	A
6.	A	18.	C	30.	D	42.	C	54.	B
7.	D	19.	B	31.	A	43.	C	55.	C
8.	D	20.	D	32.	D	44.	A	56.	A
9.	C	21.	C	33.	C	45.	C	57.	D
10.	B	22.	A	34.	A	46.	C	58.	A
11.	D	23.	A	35.	B	47.	B		
12.	A	24.	D	36.	A	48.	D		

1. **The correct answer is (A).** The product term is $\frac{1}{2} \times \frac{1}{2} = \frac{1}{4}$. Thus, $\frac{1}{4} + \frac{1}{4} = \frac{2}{4} = \frac{1}{2}$.

2. **The correct answer is (A).** Add the figures inside the parentheses and multiply by the 0.25 to get 2, then add 4 to get 6.

3. **The correct answer is (D).** Add the figures inside the parentheses and divide by 0.4 to get 30, then subtract 1 to get 29.

4. **The correct answer is (B).** The quotient of the terms in parentheses is $\frac{12}{6} = 2$, then multiply by 2.5 to get 5.

5. **The correct answer is (D).** Five to the third power $= 5^3 = 5 \times 5 \times 5 = 125$. Then, $125 + 5 = 130$.

6. **The correct answer is (A).** For the two terms, $2 \times 2 \times 2 = 8$ and $2 \times 2 = 4$. Then, $8 \times 4 = 32$.

7. **The correct answer is (D).** In general, any number raised to a negative exponent is equal to the inverse of the number raised to the corresponding positive exponent, e.g., $Y^{-2} = \frac{1}{Y^2}$.

8. **The correct answer is (D).** Solve this problem by inspection. The cube root of 8 is 2, i.e., $2 \times 2 \times 2 = 8$.

9. **The correct answer is (C).** $\sqrt{2} \times \sqrt{6} \times \sqrt{3} = \sqrt{2 \times 6 \times 3} = \sqrt{36} = 6$.

10. **The correct answer is (B).** The log of a number is the power to which the base of the log must be raised to obtain the number. Here, the base 5 must be raised to the second power to obtain 25.

11. **The correct answer is (D).** A prime number is a whole number that cannot be divided by any other whole number but itself or 1.

12. **The correct answer is (A).** The vertical bars instruct you to take the absolute (positive) value of the enclosed number. Thus, $13 - |-2| + |-6| = 13 - 2 + 6 = 17$.

13. **The correct answer is (C).** The expression illustrates different associations of the multipliers 5, 25, 8, and $(3 + 4)$.

14. **The correct answer is (D).** $\frac{12 + [15 \times 2 - 7 \times 8 + 2]}{8} = \frac{12 + [-24]}{8} = \frac{-12}{8} = \frac{-3}{2} = -1\frac{1}{2}$.

15. **The correct answer is (B).** $\frac{KL^2}{C} = 5 \times \frac{10^2}{2} = 5 \times \frac{100}{2} = 250$.

16. **The correct answer is (B).** The volume of a cylinder is obtained as the area of the circle that forms its base, πr^2, and its height, h. Cylinder volume $= \pi r^2 h$.

17. **The correct answer is (D).** Collecting terms in x on the left, $4x + 6x = 17 + 3$; $10x = 20$; $x = 2$.

18. **The correct answer is (C).** Multiply each side of the equation by the product of the denominators (lowest common denominator) to get $2(2y + 3) - 10 \times 10 = 5(4 - 3y)$, or $4y + 6 - 100 = 20 - 15y$. Collect terms in y on the left: $4y + 15y = 20 - 6 + 100$. Or, $19y = 114$, and thus $y = 6$.

19. **The correct answer is (B).** Multiply to eliminate the parentheses: $z + 5 = 4z + 8 - 2z - 1$. Collect terms in z on the left: $z - 4z + 2z = 8 - 1 - 5$, or, $-z = 2$, $z = -2$.

20. **The correct answer is (D).** One has two equations: $J = 3H$ and $J - 4 = 5(H - 4)$. Substituting the first into the second gives $3H - 4 = 5H - 20$. Thus, $-2H = -16$, or $H = 8$. Substituting this into the first equation gives $J = 3 \times 8 = 24$.

21. **The correct answer is (C).** Let the initial speed be x mph. Then, $x \times 2$ hrs. + $(x + 20) \times 4$ hrs. = 320 miles. Thus, $2x + 4x + 80 = 320$. Or, $6x = 240$ and $x = 40$.

22. **The correct answer is (A).** Collecting terms in y on the left, $5y^2 - 10y = 0$. Factoring, $5y(y-2) = 0$. Therefore, $y = 0$ and $y = 2$.

23. **The correct answer is (A).** Collecting terms in Z on the left gives: $aZ - cZ = d + b$, or, $Z(a - c) = d + b$, and $Z = \frac{d+b}{a-c}$.

24. **The correct answer is (D).** Collecting terms in A on the left: $8A - 3A > -7 + 17$, or, $5A > 10$, and $A > 2$.

25. **The correct answer is (B).** Multiply all terms by $6 \times 4 = 24$ to clear the denominators: $4B - 6B \geq 24$, so $-2B \geq 24$ and $-B \geq 12$. Multiply by -1 and reverse the inequality to get $B \leq -12$.

26. **The correct answer is (C).** Collect terms in C on the left: $3C - 8C < -3 + 18$, or $-5C < 15$ and $-C < 3$. Multiply by -1 and reverse the equality to get: $C > -3$.

27. **The correct answer is (B).** The equation can be factored to give $(y + 5)(y + 2) = 0$. Each factor can be equated to zero, thus, $y + 5 = 0$ and $y + 2 = 0$. Accordingly, the solutions are $y = -5$ and $y = -2$.

28. **The correct answer is (C).** The equation is factored. Each term can be set equal to zero. Thus, $x = 0$ and $x - 12 = 0$. The solutions are $x = 0$ and $x = 12$.

29. **The correct answer is (A).** Collecting all terms on the left: $K^2 - 5K^2 + 36 = 0$ or, $4K^2 - 36 = 0$ and $K^2 = 9$. Thus, $K = 3$ and $K = -3$.

30. **The correct answer is (D).** Adding the equations gives: $0B + 6C = 12$. Thus, $C = 2$.

31. **The correct answer is (A).** Multiply the second equation by 2 and subtract it from the first to get: $3B = -9$ or $B = -3$.

32. **The correct answer is (D).** The patient will take 3 tablets each day. Thus, x tablets is to 14 days as 3 tablets is to 1 day, i.e., $\frac{x}{14} = \frac{3}{1}$ and $x = 3 \times \frac{14}{1} = 42$.

33. **The correct answer is (C).** Let x g be the amount required to make 50 ml. Then, $\frac{x \text{ g}}{50 \text{ ml}} = \frac{16 \text{ g}}{200 \text{ ml}}$. Accordingly, $x = \frac{(50 \text{ ml} \times 16 \text{ g})}{200 \text{ ml}} = 4$ g.

34. **The correct answer is (A).** A 10 percent mixture will contain 10 g of coal tar per 100 g of the mixture. Let x g be the amount of coal tar to be mixed with 450 g of zinc oxide paste. The total weight of the mixture will be $(450 + x)$ g. Accordingly, $\frac{10 \text{ g}}{100 \text{ g}} = \frac{x \text{ g}}{(450+x)\text{g}}$.

Solve this equation for x: $10 \times (450 + x) = 100x$; $4,500 = 100x - 10x = 90x$; $x = \frac{4,500}{90} = 50$.

35. **The correct answer is (B).** The median of a set of numbers is the number in the middle when the numbers are arranged in order. Here, the ordered numbers are: 62, 72, 77, 86, 93, 96, and 98. The middle number—the fourth number—is 86.

36. The correct answer is (A). A triangle with two sides equal is an isosceles triangle with angles A and B equal. The sum of the three angles must equal $180°$, i.e., $180° = A + B + 30° = 2A + 30°$.

Or, $A = \frac{(180° - 30°)}{2} = \frac{150°}{2} = 75°$.

37. The correct answer is (C). The diagonal of a rectangle together with the sides forms a right triangle. For a right triangle, the sum of the squares of the two sides forming the right angle is equal to the square of the opposite side (here, the diagonal). Thus, $d^2 = (6 \text{ cm})^2 + (8 \text{ cm})^2 = 100 \text{ cm}^2$. Thus, $d = \sqrt{100 \text{ cm}^2} = 10$ cm.

38. The correct answer is (B). The diameter of the circle is equal to the length of the sides of the square, 8 in. The area, A, of a circle is given by $A = \pi r^2 = \pi\left[\frac{d}{2}\right]^2 = \pi\frac{d^2}{4} = 3.14 \times \frac{64}{4} = 50.2$ sq. in.

39. The correct answer is (D). Note that $\beta + 45 = 180$. Because lines A and B are parallel, $\alpha = \beta$, and thus $\alpha + 45° = 180°$. Accordingly, $\alpha = 180° - 45° = 135°$.

40. The correct answer is (B). The diagonal of the square is equal to the diameter of the circle (10). Using the Pythagorean theorem, we can obtain the length of the sides (A) of the square: $(10)^2 = A^2 + A^2 = 2A^2$, or, $A^2 = 50$. But, the area of the square is $A \times A = A^2$.

41. The correct answer is (A). The distance between two points can be obtained using the formula (derived from the Pythagorean theorem): $d = \left[(x_1 - x_2)^2 + (y_1 - y_2)^2\right]^{\frac{1}{2}}$. Here, $d = \left[(-3 - 1)^2 + (2 + 1)^2\right]^{\frac{1}{2}} = [16 + 9]^{\frac{1}{2}} = 5$.

42. The correct answer is (C). The volume of a cube will be equal to the length of a side cubed. Because the volume is 1,000, the length of each side is 10. The area of a single face is $10 \times 10 = 100$. There are six faces, thus the surface area is $6 \times 100 = 600$.

43. The correct answer is (C). The x-intercept is the value of x when $y = 0$. Thus, $0 = 5x + 25$ or $x = \frac{-25}{5} = -5$.

44. The correct answer is (A). The equation for a straight line can be obtained using the coordinates for any two points on the line. Here, we may note that at $X = 20$, $Y = 75$ and at $X = 40$, $Y = 125$. Because the slope of a straight line is constant, one can use the relationship: $\frac{(Y - Y_1)}{(X - X_1)} = \frac{(Y_2 - Y_1)}{(X_2 - X_1)}$. Putting in the values for the two points gives: $\frac{Y - 75}{X - 20} = \frac{125 - 75}{40 - 20} = \frac{50}{20}$.

Solving for Y gives $Y - 75 = (X - 20) \times \frac{50}{20}$. Or, $20Y - 1,500 = 50X - 1,000$; therefore, $Y = 2.5X + 25$.

45. The correct answer is (C). The slope of a straight line is calculated as the ratio of a segment length along the ordinate $(y_2 - y_1)$ to the corresponding segment length along the abscissa $(x_2 - x_1)$. Thus, if we take the ordinate segment to be from 50 to 150, the corresponding abscissa segment is from 1 to 3 and the ratio of their lengths is $\frac{150 - 50}{3 - 1} = \frac{100}{2} = 50$. Thus, the slope is 50, indicating a driving speed of 50 miles per hour.

46. The correct answer is (C). The equation $x^2 + y^2 = r^2$ represents a circle of radius r centered at the origin. Here, $x^2 + y^2 = 36$, thus, $r^2 = 36$, $r = 6$, and the diameter $= 2r = 12$.

47. The correct answer is (B). Here, $f(6) = 2 \times 6^3 + 5 \times 6^2 + 15 = 432 + 180 + 15 = 627$.

48. The correct answer is (D). Taking the limit of a function for a specified value of the variable corresponds to evaluating the function as the variable. Here x gets arbitrarily close to that value. Replacing x by 5 gives $\frac{25 + 6}{1} = 31$.

49. **The correct answer is (A).** Differentiating term by term, $\frac{dy}{dx} = 12x - 8 + 0 = 12x - 8$.

50. **The correct answer is (D).** Differentiating, $\frac{dy}{dx} = 3x^2 + 4x$. At $x = 5$, $\frac{dy}{dx} = 75 + 20 = 95$.

51. **The correct answer is (A).** Differentiating, $\frac{dy}{dx} = 3(x^2 + 5)^2(2x) = 6x(x^2 + 5)^2$.

52. **The correct answer is (B).**

$y = \sqrt{x-5} = (x-5)^{\frac{1}{2}}$.

Differentiating, $\frac{dy}{dx} = \left(\frac{1}{2}\right)(x-5)^{\frac{-1}{2}} = \frac{1}{(2\sqrt{x-5})}$.

53. **The correct answer is (A).** Differentiating, $dy = d(\sin 2x) + d(\cos^2 3x) = 2(\cos 2x)dx + 2(\cos 3x)d(\cos 3x) = 2(\cos 2x)dx + 2(\cos 3x)(3)(-\sin 3x)dx$. Thus, $\frac{dy}{dx} = 2(\cos 2x) - 6(\cos 3x)(\sin 3x)$.

54. **The correct answer is (B).** The goal is to find the most general function whose derivative is the integrand. This is: $6\left(\frac{1}{3}\right)x^3 + C = 2x^3 + C$ where C is an arbitrary constant.

55. **The correct answer is (C).** The general function whose derivative gives the integrand is: $4\left(\frac{1}{4}\right)x^4 - 6\left(\frac{1}{2}\right)x^2 + C = x^4 - 3x^2 + C$.

56. **The correct answer is (A).** The general function whose derivative is the integrand is: $3(-\cos x) + C = -3\cos x + C$.

57. **The correct answer is (D).** The function whose derivative gives the integrand is: $9\left(\frac{1}{3}\right)x^3 = 3x^3$. This function is evaluated at the limits of 8 and 2, i.e., $3x^3 \Big]_2^8 = 3(8)^3 - 3(2)^3 = 1512$.

58. **The correct answer is (A).** The area under the curve between 0 and 1 is given by $\int_0^1 (x^2 - 2x + 5)dx$. The function whose derivative gives the integrand is $\left(\frac{1}{3}\right)x^3 - \left(\frac{2}{2}\right)x^2 + 5x$. Evaluating between the integration limits of 0 and 1 gives:

$\left(\frac{1}{3}\right)x^3 - 2\left(\frac{1}{2}\right)x^2 + 5x \Big]_0^1 =$

$\left(\frac{1}{3}\right)(1-0) - 1(1-0) + 5(1-0) = \left(\frac{1}{3}\right) + 4 = \frac{13}{3}$.

answers

Chemistry

1.	C	13.	B	25.	D	37.	D	49.	D
2.	D	14.	A	26.	D	38.	A	50.	C
3.	B	15.	D	27.	C	39.	C	51.	B
4.	C	16.	B	28.	D	40.	D	52.	A
5.	A	17.	C	29.	B	41.	B	53.	C
6.	D	18.	B	30.	A	42.	C	54.	B
7.	C	19.	A	31.	C	43.	D	55.	D
8.	A	20.	A	32.	B	44.	A	56.	C
9.	C	21.	D	33.	A	45.	B	57.	A
10.	A	22.	B	34.	B	46.	A	58.	B
11.	D	23.	C	35.	D	47.	B		
12.	C	24.	A	36.	B	48.	D		

1. **The correct answer is (C).** nM is a short notation for nanomolarity, and it equals to 10^{-9} M. 10^{-3} M equals to 1 mM, 10^{-6} M equals to 1 mM, and 10^{-12} M equals to 1 pM.

2. **The correct answer is (D).** The mole molecular weight of NaOH is 40; therefore, 1 mol of NaOH weighs 40 g. The solution contains $0.5 \, l \times \frac{0.3 \, mol}{1} = 0.15$ mol NaOH, and the amount of NaOH needed is $0.15 \, mol \times \frac{40 \, g}{mol} = 6$ g.

3. **The correct answer is (B).** Total amount of NaCl in the final solution equals to $0.5 \, l \times \frac{1 \, mol}{1} + 0.2 \, l \times \frac{2 \, mol}{1} = 0.9$ mol; therefore, the final concentration will be $\frac{0.9 \, mol}{2 \, l} = 0.45$ M.

4. **The correct answer is (C).** An acidic solution has pH < 7, whereas a basic solution has pH > 7. When pH = 7, the solution is neutral.

5. **The correct answer is (A).** For an addition or a subtraction, the result should have the same precision as the *least* precise measurement. The number with greatest uncertainty is 10.3; therefore, the answer should be rounded to the nearest tenth, 14.8. For multiplication or division, the answer must contain the same number of significant figures as in the measurement that has the least number of significant figures.

6. **The correct answer is (D).** For a neutral atom, the number of electrons must equal to the number of protons. The number of neutrons only affects the mass of the atom but does not have direct relationship to the number of electrons.

7. **The correct answer is (C).** Isotopes only differ in their mass—they have the same number of protons and electrons. The isotopes of an element have the same chemical properties, and this is the base for isotope labeling widely used in chemistry and biological researches.

8. **The correct answer is (A).** The hydrocarbon containing seven carbon atoms is called heptane. Pentane contains 5 carbons, octane contains 8 carbons, and decane contains 10 carbons.

9. **The correct answer is (C).** The two carbons in ethylene are connected by a double bond that cannot freely rotate. The carbon has sp^2 hybrid orbitals, which is planar in geometry.

10. **The correct answer is (A).** Methlyene group is CH_2 and methine group is CH. Methane is the simplest hydrocarbon molecule.

11. **The correct answer is (D).** R from the Latin *rectus* meaning right and S from the Latin *sinister*, meaning left. R and S are used to assign the absolute configuration of chiral centers in a molecule.

12. **The correct answer is (C).** Both oxygen and nitrogen have sp^3 hybrid orbitals. Oxygen in water molecule has two lone pairs to occupy the remaining two oribitals. Nitrogen atom in ammonia has one lone pair.

13. **The correct answer is (B).** There are two hydrogen atoms in H_2O_2. The molecular weight of H_2O_2 is 34; therefore, the percent composition by mass for hydrogen is $\frac{2}{34} = 0.059 = 5.9\%$.

14. **The correct answer is (A).** Chlorous acid is $HClO_2$, chloric acid is $HClO_3$, and perchloric acid is $HClO_4$.

15. **The correct answer is (D).** A chemical equation must obey the law of conservation of matter. The number of atoms in reactants must equal the number of atoms in the product. The number of oxygen atoms is not balanced in choices (A) and (B). The numbers of K and Cl are not balanced in choice (C). Only in choice (D) are all the atoms balanced properly.

16. **The correct answer is (B).** Strong acids, strong bases, and ionic salts are all strong electrolytes. Weak acids and weak bases are normally weak electrolytes. Acetic acid is a weak acid.

17. **The correct answer is (C).** Brønsted acid is a proton donor, and Brønsted base is a proton acceptor. $H_2PO_4^-$ can accept a proton to become H_3PO_4 or release a proton to become HPO_4^{2-}. Therefore, it can act as either an acid or a base.

18. **The correct answer is (B).** Ca gives up electrons to oxygen in the reaction; therefore, it is a reducing agent. Oxygen gains electrons in the reaction, and its oxidation number changed from 0 to −2. The product is solid CaO, which has much lower entropy than the gaseous oxygen.

19. **The correct answer is (A).** One atm and 0°C is the standard condition, at which 1 mole of gas occupies 22.4 liters of volume. One gram of hydrogen gas is 0.5mol; therefore, the volume it occupies at standard condition is 11.2 l.

20. **The correct answer is (A).** It tests the understanding of Graham's law of effusion: The rates of effusion of two gases at the same temperature and pressure are inversely proportional to the square roots of their densities or molar masses. Oxygen has a larger molar mass than nitrogen; therefore, nitrogen has a higher effusion rate.

21. **The correct answer is (D).** For principle quantum number n, the maximum number of electrons that can be present is $2n^2$. For $n = 2$, this is 8.

22. **The correct answer is (B).** Pauli exclusion principle.

23. **The correct answer is (C).** The nitrogen atoms in NH_3 has sp^3 hybrid orbital, thus NH_3 is tetrahedral in geometry with a lone pair occupies one corner. All other molecules in the choice have planar geometry.

24. **The correct answer is (A).** Choices (B) and (C) have a carbonyl group that contains a pi bond. Naphthalene is a fused-ring aromatic hydrocarbon that contains a pi bond. Only CH_3OH does not contain any pi bond.

25. **The correct answer is (D).** A hydrogen bond is a chemical bond that is formed between polar molecules that contain hydrogen covalently bonded to a small, highly electronegative atom, such as fluorine, oxygen, or nitrogen. Carbon usually cannot form hydrogen bond due to its low electronegative property.

26. The correct answer is (D). Two acetic acid molecules can form a dimer via hydrogen bonding. This dimer is much less polar compared with a single acetic acid molecule; hence, it is soluble to nonpolar solvents. It is not an aromatic compound, nor can it react with benzene under normal conditions.

27. The correct answer is (C). The *homolysis* process is based on osmosis, in which water diffuses from a dilute solution or water through a semipermeable membrane into a solution of higher concentration. Because water moves into the cell, the solution is more dilute than that inside the cell; therefore, it is a *hypotonic* solution. A *hypertonic* solution has a higher concentration, whereas an isotonic solution has equal concentration compared with that of the other side of the semipermeable membrane.

28. The correct answer is (D). K_w is essentially an equilibrium constant; therefore, it is dependent on temperature. It does not depend on the pH (which indicates the concentration of proton) of the solution. It does not depend on pressure because the system is in solution state.

29. The correct answer is (B). At 25°C, pH + pOH = pK_w = 14; hence, pOH =10, and $[OH^-] = 10^{-10}$M.

30. The correct answer is (A). The *stronger* the acid is, the *weaker* its conjugate base.

31. The correct answer is (C). CaO forms base $Ca(OH)_2$ with water. All others form acids when they react with water.

32. The correct answer is (B). The maximum possible concentration of $[H^+]$ in a 0.1 M solution of HA is 0.1 M. For strong acid, this is true. For weak acid, the $[H^+]$ is much less than 0.1 M because of incomplete dissociation. Therefore, the pH is larger than 1.

33. The correct answer is (A). The solution is basic. This salt is formed by a weak acid HCN with a weak base NH_3. Both of the anion (CN^-) and cation ($NH4^+$) will undergo hydrolysis in water. Since K_b >> K_a, the anion hydrolysis that produces $[OH^-]$ will be more extensive than the cation hydrolysis that produces $[H_3O^+]$.

34. The correct answer is (B). A buffer solution is a solution of a weak acid or base and its salt. $HClO_4$ is a very strong acid—hence, this acid and its salt cannot make a buffer system.

35. The correct answer is (D). When water vapor becomes water, the water molecules are more ordered. Since entropy is a direct measure of the randomness or disorder of a system, for the same molar amount of substance, it is always true that $S_{solid} < S_{liquid} << S_{gas}$.

36. The correct answer is (B). Mercury has both +1 (mercurous) and +2 (mercuric) oxidation numbers in its compounds.

37. The correct answer is (D). Fluorine is an exception because it is the most electronegative element. It can only have two oxidation numbers, 0 (as in F_2) and −1, in its compounds.

38. The correct answer is (A). Hydrogen peroxide is not a planar molecule. Since it can form hydrogen bonding with water, it is easily miscible with water. The oxidation number is −1 in hydrogen peroxide, in the middle of −2 (such as in MgO) and 0 (in O_2); hence, it can act as either an oxidation or a reducing agent.

39. **The correct answer is (C).** The atomic mass does not change, so only an electron is emitted.

40. **The correct answer is (D).** Atoms in triple bonds are fixed with the pi bonds and are not allowed to freely rotate.

41. **The correct answer is (B).** The three structural isomers are: $CH_3CH_2CH_2CH_2CH_3$, $CH_3CH_2CH(CH_3)_2$, and $C(CH_3)_4$.

42. **The correct answer is (C).** *R*- and *S*- are used to assign absolute configuration in chiral atoms in a molecule. *Ortho*- and *para*- are used for positions in aromatic rings, and *n*- and *t*- are used for hydrocarbon branching.

43. **The correct answer is (D).** It does not have the general ester functional group of RCOOR´.

44. **The correct answer is (A).** H_2S is hydrogen sulfide. Choices (C) and (D) do not exist.

45. **The correct answer is (B).** Avogadro's law and Boyle's law have nothing to do with chemical reaction mechanisms, whereas Saytzeff's rule deals with dehydration.

46. **The correct answer is (A).** The oxidation state of carbon is 4 in CO_2, –2 in CH_3OH, 2 in HCOOH, and 0 in CH_4, respectively.

47. **The correct answer is (B).** The –OH group from the carboxylic acid and the –H in hydroxyl group of the alcohol form water molecules in the esterification reaction.

48. **The correct answer is (D).** Phenol is a stronger acid than methanol because of the stabilization effect from the aromatic ring when it loses a proton. However, it is not as acidic as acetic acid.

49. **The correct answer is (D).** Tollen's test for aldehydes is based on the ability of silver ions to oxidize aldehydes. Ketones, esters, and amines cannot be oxidized under this condition.

50. **The correct answer is (C).** The maximum number of possible stereoisomers is 2^n, where *n* is the number of nonidentical asymmetric carbon atoms.

51. **The correct answer is (B).** Sucrose is sweeter than glucose. Glucose contains asymmetric carbons and it is optically active. It contains aldehyde group; hence, it gives positive Tollen's test and can be reduced to alcohol by hydrogen.

52. **The correct answer is (A).** Amino acids have the general formula of $RCHNH_2COOH$. They can be classified as neutral amino acids when their molecules have the same number of amino and carboxyl groups, as acids when their molecules have more carboxyl groups than amino groups, or as basic when their molecules have more amino groups than carboxyl groups. In the choices given, only glycine has the same number of carboxyl and amino group. Lysine, arginine, and histidine all have more extra amino groups and are classified as basic amino acids.

53. **The correct answer is (C).** Amides have the general formula of $R-CO-NH_2$, and the $-NH_2$ can be –NHR or $-NR_2$. $R-CO-NR_3$ has an extra R group attached to the nitrogen.

54. The correct answer is (B). Trichlorbenzene can have three isomers, 1, 2, 3–; 1, 2, 4–; and 1, 3, 5–trichlorbenzene. Another arrangement is essentially equivalent to one of these three isomers.

55. The correct answer is (D). Diels–Alder reaction is the addition of an alkene (which is called the dienophile) to a diene to form a cyclohexene. It is the most important cycloaddition reaction from the point of view of synthesis. A carboxylic acid and an alcohol can react to form an ester; an alkene and a halogen can have addition reaction; an acid and a base is an acid–base neutralization reaction.

56. The correct answer is (C). Fatty acids and steroids belong to *lipids*. Cholesterols belong to *steroids*. Starch, however, belongs to *carbohydrates*, not lipids.

57. The correct answer is (A). A primary amine has the general formula of RNH_2, a secondary amine has the general formula of R_2NH, and a tertiary amine has the general formula of R_3N.

58. The correct answer is (B). The α-helix and β-sheet are two examples of protein secondary structure. The primary structure of a protein refers to the number, kind, and sequences of amino acid units comprising the polypeptide chain or chains. The secondary structure refers to the regular, three-dimensional structure held together by hydrogen bonding between the carbonyl oxygen and the amino hydrogen in the polypeptide chains. The tertiary structure normally refers to the overall shape of a protein.

Verbal Ability

1.	A	13.	A	25.	A	37.	C	49.	A
2.	D	14.	B	26.	D	38.	C	50.	B
3.	C	15.	A	27.	D	39.	D	51.	D
4.	A	16.	D	28.	B	40.	B	52.	B
5.	D	17.	D	29.	C	41.	C	53.	D
6.	A	18.	A	30.	A	42.	B	54.	A
7.	B	19.	B	31.	B	43.	D	55.	A
8.	A	20.	C	32.	D	44.	A	56.	D
9.	C	21.	D	33.	B	45.	D	57.	B
10.	A	22.	A	34.	A	46.	D	58.	D
11.	D	23.	A	35.	C	47.	C		
12.	A	24.	B	36.	B	48.	D		

1. **The correct answer is (A).** APPLAUD-ING (v.)—expressing approval of or praising. *Adulating* (v.)—praising or admiring excessively.

2. **The correct answer is (D).** DIVORCE (n.)—the action or an instance of legally dissolving a marriage. *Sunder* (v.)—to break or wrench apart; sever.

3. **The correct answer is (C).** PHARMA-CIST (n.)—a person trained in pharmacy. *Apothecary* (n.)—one who prepares and sells drugs or compounds for medicinal purposes.

4. **The correct answer is (A).** DOCK (n.)—the area of water between two piers or alongside a pier that receives a ship for loading, unloading, or repairs. *Pier* (n.)—a platform extending from a shore over water and supported by piles or pillars.

5. **The correct answer is (D).** RESULT (n.)—the consequence of a particular action. *Sequence* (n.)—a following of one thing after another.

6. **The correct answer is (A).** FERTILE (adj.)—capable of initiating, sustaining, or supporting reproduction. *Fecund* (adj.)—capable of producing offspring or vegetation.

7. **The correct answer is (B).** AUBERGE (n.)—an establishment for the lodging and entertaining of travelers. *Caravansary* (n.)—an inn surrounding a court in eastern countries where caravans of people rest at night.

8. **The correct answer is (A).** DEAN (n.)—the head of a division, faculty, college, or school of a university. *Leader* (n.)—one who leads or guides.

9. **The correct answer is (C).** ENGAGING (adv.)—holding the attention of. *Loathsome* (adj.)—offensive or disgusting.

10. **The correct answer is (A).** WALL-FLOWER (n.)—one who does not participate in the activity at a social event because of shyness or unpopularity. *Dancer* (n.)—a person engaged in or performing a dance.

11. **The correct answer is (D).** JOHN DORY (n.)—a North Atlantic fish with a laterally compressed body and long spines on the dorsal fin. *Fish* (n.)—an aquatic animal.

12. **The correct answer is (A).** MENIAL (n.)—a person doing menial work, specifically a domestic servant. *Dray horse* (n.)—a horse adapted for drawing heavy loads.

13. **The correct answer is (A).** AGREE-MENT (n.)—harmony of opinion or accord. *Contract* (n.)—the writing or document containing an agreement.

14. **The correct answer is (B).** VORTEX (n.)—a spiral motion of fluid within a limited area. *Maelstrom* (n.)—a whirlpool of extraordinary size or violence.

15. **The correct answer is (A).** WAGGLE (v.)—to move frequently one way and the other. *Switch* (v.)—a shift from one to another.

16. **The correct answer is (D).** LIAR (n.)—one who tells lies. *Perjurer* (n.)—a person who deliberately gives false testimony.

17. **The correct answer is (D).** TACKY (adj.)—lacking style or good taste. *Modish* (adj.)—fashionable or stylish.

18. **The correct answer is (A).** WRECK-AGE (n.)—the act of wrecking or the state of being wrecked. *Sabotage* (n.)—destruction of property or obstruction of normal operations.

19. **The correct answer is (B).** THESPIAN (n.)—an actor or actress. *Mummer* (n.)—a performer or actor in a pantomime.

20. **The correct answer is (C).** ANNIHI-LATE (v.)—to destroy completely. *Invent* (v.)—to produce or contrive by the use of ingenuity or imagination.

21. **The correct answer is (D).** HARE (n.)—any of various swift long-eared lagomorph mammals. *Slowpoke* (n.)—one that moves, works, or acts slowly.

22. **The correct answer is (A).** RECREANT (adj.)—unfaithful or disloyal to a belief, duty, or cause. *Perfidious* (adj.)—of, relating to, or marked by perfidy; treacherous.

23. **The correct answer is (A).** POLITY (n.)—the form of government of a nation, state, church, or organization. *Course* (n.)—the act or action of moving in a path from point to point.

24. **The correct answer is (B).** IRASCIBLE (adj.)—marked by hot temper and easily provoked anger. *Tolerant* (adj.)—inclined to bear or put up with.

25. **The correct answer is (A).** HORRID (adj.)—causing horror; dreadful. *Lurid* (adj.)—causing shock or horror; gruesome.

26. **The correct answer is (D).** "Balmy" and "mild" are synonyms. Therefore, the task is to look for a synonym for "faithful," which in this case is "staunch."

27. **The correct answer is (D).** "Hope" and "despondency" are contrasting concepts. The concept that contrasts with "pleasure" is "anguish."

28. **The correct answer is (B).** A "scepter" is a symbol of "authority;" "scales" are symbols of "justice."

29. **The correct answer is (C).** This a whole-to-part analogy. An "archipelago" is made up of "islands"; a "galaxy" is made up of "stars." A "galaxy" is part of the "universe"; the order of the relationship is the reverse of that between "archipelago" and "island." "The Milky Way" is a "galaxy."

30. **The correct answer is (A).** In this analogy of degree, a "feast" is a rich and expensive "meal"; "vellum" is a rich and expensive kind of "paper."

31. **The correct answer is (B).** The relationship is one of degree. A "leap" is a very large "jump"; a "stride" is a very large "step."

32. **The correct answer is (D).** This is an analogy not of true synonyms but of synonyms as used in common parlance. Thus "turn on a light" is used interchangeably with "turn on a lamp," and "have a seat" is used interchangeable with "have a chair."

33. **The correct answer is (B).** "Abundance" and "dearth" are antonyms. The

opposite of "abrogate" (to nullify or cancel) is "establish."

34. **The correct answer is (A).** This is a descriptive analogy. A "pound" is a measurement of "weight." Likewise, a "kilogram" is sometimes considered a measure of weight but is also a measure of "mass."

35. **The correct answer is (C).** The relationship is one of measurement. A "division" of a baseball game is an "inning"; an "era" is a phase of "history."

36. **The correct answer is (B).** The correspondence is one of object to action. One may "exorcise evil"; one may "break bread."

37. **The correct answer is (C).** In this cause-and-effect analogy, one effect of excessive "wind" is soil "erosion"; an effect of an excessive "deficit" is "borrowing" to make up for expenditures. Excessive spending is a cause of a deficit, not an effect.

38. **The correct answer is (C).** The relationship is one of origin or sequence. A "raisin" is a dried "grape," just as a "prune" is a dried "plum."

39. **The correct answer is (D).** A "safe" is opened by a "combination"; a "necklace" is opened by a "clasp."

40. **The correct answer is (B).** "Binding" secures or holds a "book" together; "welding" secures or holds a "tank" together.

41. **The correct answer is (C).** "Eminent" and "lowly" are antonyms; "frequent" and "rare" are antonyms.

42. **The correct answer is (B).** On two blank questions, it's easiest to consider one blank at a time. Attacking the second blank first makes the most sense since you know that it is in contrast to minor points (the trigger word "Although" should be your clue.) What is a contrast to a minor point? A major one. You should

go look for something like major or important. That eliminates (A) and (C). Of the remaining choices, "debate" fits best into the first blank, as a debate is more likely to have "themes" than is an agreement or discovery.

43. **The correct answer is (D).** The blank is a word that goes along with "created excitement" so it is definitely positive. "Engendered" is a positive verb that flows with greater interest.

44. **The correct answer is (A).** The "Although" at the beginning of the sentence clues you into the fact that this is a contrast sentence. The good times spoken of in the present are contrasted with what is in the blank. What is a contrast with good times? Tough or "leaner" times.

45. **The correct answer is (D).** The second blank is a positive word since the logic of the sentence is that "though" the early theories were "crude," they were still helpful.

46. **The correct answer is (D).** Here the first blank seems more assailable. You know that it has to pair with "factually misleading." As for the second blank, you know two things: it pairs with "superior mastery of language," and it "masks" the "problems" mentioned in the first part of the sentence. Thus, it must be something very positive.

47. **The correct answer is (C).** The second blank requires a word meaning "to understand." "Grasp" fits well. The first blank goes along with the professor being "visibly frustrated."

48. **The correct answer is (D).** The word "but" in the sentence is the key clue. It tells you that the first and second parts of the sentence are in contrast to each other. In the first part we are told that Mr. Thomas had earned the reputation as a "miser," and so in the second part you should expect to find a strong contrast to this.

49. The correct answer is (A). Consider the first blank first. "Shifts" in the "demographics" of a country would at least challenge "traditional political alliances" and at most destroy them. Since the sentence speaks of "nascent political parties," you can infer that the traditional ones are at least being challenged. "Solvent" and "elusive" are not good answer choices for the first blank. As the old political parties are being challenged, the new ones then are gaining ground. Between "procure" and "secure," "secure" is the better choice since "procure" intimates buying, and one does not purchase "large swathes of the electoral landscape."

50. The correct answer is (B). What is a word that goes with "public" and "can be persuaded"? "Opinion." The word "ostensibly" clues you to the fact that the second blank is a strong contrast to "process of popular persuasion."

51. The correct answer is (D). You are looking for a word that modifies "feuds between rival factions" of a company. "Internecine" means fighting within a group and is the best choice.

52. The correct answer is (B). The sentence tells us that the first blank can be described as the practice of appointing "friends and associates to high posts." The second blank is a contrast to the first since the favoritism of the "predecessors" is being "eschewed" in favor of the new way. "Merit" makes more sense than "work."

53. The correct answer is (D). In this sentence, the author's customary style of correspondence is being contrasted with the style in her most recent letter. "Customarily" her style is "deliberate," but in this letter it is "convoluted." Therefore, in the first blank, you are looking for a word that pairs well with "deliberate" and contrasts well with "convoluted." In the second blank, you are looking for a word that pairs well with "convoluted" and contrasts well with "deliberate."

54. The correct answer is (A). A "successful demolition" crew demolishes buildings. "Raze" means to destroy completely.

55. The correct answer is (A). Something like "punishable" or "responsible" works well. "Culpable" is the best fit.

56. The correct answer is (D). The first blank is clearly a negative term since "publicity surrounding mismanagement" would hurt a "company's credibility." In the second blank, we can infer that it must be positive since it is on its account that the company "remained solvent."

57. The correct answer is (B). The "Though" at the beginning of the sentence clues you into the fact that the official's hopes were not achieved. Thus, his assurances must not have had their desired effect. Assurances are meant to "calm," so "assuage" is the best choice.

58. The correct answer is (D). The sentence structure indicates that the word in the blank is described by the "younger sibling . . . taking on mannerisms. . . ." What are the younger siblings doing? They are "copying" their older siblings.

Critical Thinking Essay

Have someone you respect—a professor or a professional writer—read your essay. Then ask him or her to grade it based on the following scoring criteria:

SCORE POINT 5—SUPERIOR

The writer is in command of the conventions of language; makes very few, if any, mistakes in sentence formation, usage, and mechanics. Some evidence is shown of advanced or innovative techniques.

SCORE POINT 4—EFFECTIVE

On the whole, the writer correctly applies the conventions of language, though there are some mistakes in sentence formation, usage, or mechanics. However, none of these errors are serious enough to interfere with the overall flow of the response or with its meaning.

SCORE POINT 3—ADEQUATE

The writer is fairly successful in applying the conventions of language. Several mistakes in sentence formation, usage, or mechanics are present. While the density of these errors may interfere with the overall flow of the response, they do not interfere with its meaning.

SCORE POINT 2—MARGINAL

The writer is marginally successful in applying the conventions of language. Patterns of mistakes in sentence formation, usage, and mechanics significantly detract from the presentation. At times the meaning of the response may be weakened.

SCORE POINT 1—WEAK

The writer's achievement in applying the conventions of language is limited. Frequent and serious mistakes in sentence formation, usage, and mechanics make the response difficult to understand.

APPENDIXES

APPENDIX A   AACP Member Colleges and
            Schools of Pharmacy

APPENDIX B   State Boards of Pharmacy

APPENDIX C   Licensure Requirements

AACP Member Colleges and Schools of Pharmacy

ALABAMA

Harrison School of Pharmacy
Auburn University
217 Walker Building
Auburn, AL 36849-5501
Phone: (334) 844-8348
Web site: www.pharmacy.auburn.edu

McWhorter School of Pharmacy
Samford University
800 Lakeshore Drive
Birmingham, AL 35229-7027
Phone: (205) 726-2820
Web site: www.samford.edu/schools/ pharmacy.html

ARIZONA

College of Pharmacy
Glendale Midwestern University
19555 North 59th Avenue
Glendale, AZ 85308
Phone: (623) 572-3500
Web site: www.midwestern.edu/cpg

College of Pharmacy
The University of Arizona
1703 East Mabel
P.O. Box 210207
Tucson, AZ 85721
Phone: (520) 626-1427
Web site: www.pharmacy.arizona.edu

appendix A

ARKANSAS

College of Pharmacy
University of Arkansas for Medical Sciences
4301 West Markham - Slot 522
Little Rock, AR 72205-7122
Phone: (501) 686-5557
Web site: www.uams.edu/cop

CALIFORNIA

School of Pharmacy
Loma Linda University
West Hall
Loma Linda, CA 92350
Phone: (909) 558-1300
Web site: www.llu.edu/llu/sps/index.html

School of Pharmacy and Pharmaceutical Sciences
University of California, San Diego
9500 Gelman Drive
San Diego, CA 92093-0657
Phone: (858) 822-4900
Web site: www.pharmacy.ucsd.edu

School of Pharmacy
University of California at San Francisco
521 Parnassus Avenue, Clinical Sciences Room C-156
San Francisco, CA 94143
Phone: (415) 476-2733
Web site: www.pharmacy.ucsf.edu

Thomas J. Long School of Pharmacy & Health Sciences
University of the Pacific
3601 Pacific Avenue
Stockton, CA 95211
Phone: (209) 946-2561
Web site: www1.uop.edu/pharmacy/ index.html

School of Pharmacy
University of Southern California
1985 Zonal Avenue
Los Angeles, CA 90089-9121
Phone: (323) 442-1369
Web site: usc.edu/schools/pharmacy

College of Pharmacy
Western University of Health Sciences
College Plaza
309 East Second Street
Pomona, CA 91766-1854
Phone: (909) 469-5500
Web site: www.westernu.edu/xp/edu/pharmacy/home.xml

COLORADO

School of Pharmacy
University of Colorado Health Sciences Center
C238 4
200 East Ninth Avenue
Denver, CO 80262
Phone: (303) 315-5055
Web site: www.uchsc.edu/sop

CONNECTICUT

School of Pharmacy
The University of Connecticut
372 Fairfield Road
Unit 2092
Storrs, CT 06269-2092
Phone: (860) 486-2129
Web site: www.pharmacy.uconn.edu

DISTRICT OF COLUMBIA

School of Pharmacy
Howard University College of Pharmacy, Nursing & AHS
2300 4th Street NW
Washington, DC 20059
Phone: (202) 806-6530
Web site: www.cpnahs.howard.edu

FLORIDA

College of Pharmacy and Pharmaceutical Sciences
Florida Agricultural and Mechanical University
201 Dyson Pharmacy Building
Tallahassee, FL 32307-3800
Phone: (850) 599-3301
Web site: www.168.223.36.3/acad/colleges/copps

College of Pharmacy
Nova Southeastern University Health Professions Division
3200 South University Drive
Fort Lauderdale, FL 33328
Phone: (954) 262-1300
Web site: www.pharmacy.nova.edu

School of Pharmacy
Palm Beach Atlantic University
901 South Flagler Drive
West Palm Beach, FL 33416
Phone: (561) 803-2700
Web site: www.cosmas.pbac.edu/pharmacy

College of Pharmacy
University of Florida
P.O. Box 100484, JHMHC
101 South Newell Drive, #4334
Gainesville, FL 32611
Phone: (352) 273-6601
Web site: www.cop.ufl.edu

GEORGIA

Southern School of Pharmacy
Mercer University
3001 Mercer University Drive
Atlanta, GA 30341-4155
Phone: (678) 547-6304
Web site: www.mercer.edu/pharmacy

School of Pharmacy
South University
709 Mall Boulevard
Savannah, GA 31406
Phone: (912) 201-8123
Web site: www.southuniversity.edu

College of Pharmacy
The University of Georgia
D.W. Brooks Drive
Athens, GA 30602
Phone: (706) 542-1911
Web site: www.rx.uga.edu

IDAHO

College of Pharmacy
Idaho State University
P.O. Box 8288
970 South 5th Avenue
Pocatello, ID 83209-8288
Phone: (208) 282-2175
Web site: www.pharmacy.isu.edu

ILLINOIS

Chicago College of Pharmacy
Midwestern University
555 31st Street
Downers Grove, IL 60515-1235
Phone: (630) 971-6417
Web site: www.midwestern.edu/pages/ccp.html

College of Pharmacy (M/C 874)
University of Illinois at Chicago
833 South Wood Street, Suite 145
Chicago, IL 60612
Phone: (312) 996-7240
Web site: www.uic.edu/pharmacy

INDIANA

College of Pharmacy and Health Sciences
Butler University
4600 Sunset Avenue
Indianapolis, IN 46208-3485
Phone: (317) 940-9322
Web site: www.butler.edu/cophs

School of Pharmacy and Pharmacal Sciences
Purdue University
1330 Heine Pharmacy Building
West Lafayette, IN 47907-1330
Phone: (765) 494-1368
Web site: www.pharmacy.purdue.edu

IOWA

College of Pharmacy and Health Sciences
Drake University
2507 University Avenue
Des Moines, IA 50311-4505
Phone: (515) 271-2172
Web site: www.pharmacy.drake.edu

College of Pharmacy
The University of Iowa
115 South Grand Avenue
Iowa City, IA 52242
Phone: (319) 335-8794
Web site: www.pharmacy.uiowa.edu

KANSAS

School of Pharmacy
University of Kansas
1251 Wescoe Hall Drive
Malott Hall #2056
Lawrence, KS 66045-7582
Phone: (785) 864-3591
Web site: www.pharm.ukans.edu/dean/ index.htm

KENTUCKY

College of Pharmacy
University of Kentucky
Rose Street—Pharmacy Building
Lexington, KY 40536-0082
Phone: (859) 323-7601
Web site: www.mc.uky.edu/Pharmacy

LOUISIANA

College of Health Sciences
The University of Louisiana at Monroe
700 University Avenue
Monroe, LA 71209-0400
Phone: (318) 342-1600
Web site: www.rxweb.ulm.edu/pharmacy

College of Pharmacy
Xavier University of Louisiana
1 Drexel Drive
New Orleans, LA 70125-1098
Phone: 504-483-7500
Web site: www.xula.edu/pharmacy

MARYLAND

School of Pharmacy
University of Maryland
20 North Pine Street
Baltimore, MD 21201-1180
Phone: (410) 706-8546
Web site: www.pharmacy.umaryland.edu

MASSACHUSETTS

School of Pharmacy
Boston Massachusetts College of Pharmacy and Health Sciences
179 Longwood Avenue
Boston, MA 02115-5896
Phone: (617) 732-2781
Web site: www.mcp.edu

School of Pharmacy
Worcester Massachusetts College of Pharmacy and Health Sciences
19 Foster Street
Worcester, MA 01608
Phone: (508) 890-8855
Web site: www.mcp.edu

School of Pharmacy
Bouve College of Health Sciences
Northeastern University
206 Mugar Hall
Boston, MA 02115
Phone: (617) 373-3380
Web site: www.neu.edu/bouve/pharma.html

MICHIGAN

College of Pharmacy
Ferris State University
220 Ferris Drive
Big Rapids, MI 49307-2740
Phone: (231) 591-2254
Web site: www.ferris.edu/htmls/colleges/ pharmacy

College of Pharmacy
The University of Michigan
428 Church Street
Ann Arbor, MI 48109-1065
Phone: (734) 764-7312
Web site: www.umich.edu/~pharmacy

Eugene Applebaum College of Pharmacy & Health Sciences
Wayne State University
259 Mack Avenue
Detroit, MI 48201-2417
Phone: (313) 577-1574
Web site: www.cphs.wayne.edu/index.htm

MINNESOTA

College of Pharmacy
University of Minnesota
5-130 Weaver—Densford Hall
308 Harvard Street SE
Minneapolis, MN 55455-0343
Phone: (612) 624-1900
Web site: www.pharmacy.umn.edu

College of Pharmacy
Duluth University of Minnesota
Kirby Plaza
1208 Kirby Drive
Room 386
Duluth, MN 55812-2496
Phone: (218) 726-6000

MISSISSIPPI

School of Pharmacy
The University of Mississippi
Thad Cochran Research Center
Room 1026
P.O. Box 1848
University, MS 38655-1848
Phone: (662) 915-7265
Web site: www.olemiss.edu/depts/pharm_school

MISSOURI

St. Louis College of Pharmacy
4588 Parkview Place
St. Louis, MO 63110-1088
Phone: (314) 446-8000
Web site: www.stlcop.edu

School of Pharmacy
University of Missouri—Kansas City
5005 Rockhill Road
Kansas City, MO 64110-2499
Phone: (816) 235-1609
Web site: www.umkc.edu/pharmacy

MONTANA

School of Pharmacy and Allied Health Sciences
The University of Montana
32 Campus Drive #1512
Missoula, MT 59812-1512
Phone: (406) 243-4621
Web site: www.umt.edu/pharmacy

NEBRASKA

School of Pharmacy and Health Professions
Creighton University
2500 California Plaza
Omaha, NE 68178-0104
Phone: (402) 280-2950
Web site: www.pharmacy.creighton.edu

College of Pharmacy
University of Nebraska
986000 Nebraska Medical Center
Omaha, NE 68198
Phone: (402) 559-4333
Web site: www.unmc.edu/pharmacy

NEVADA

Nevada College of Pharmacy
11 Sunset Way
Henderson, NV 89014-2333
Phone: (702) 990-4433
Web site: www.nvcp.edu

NEW JERSEY

Ernest Mario School of Pharmacy
Rutgers, the State University of New Jersey
160 Frelinghuysen Road
Piscataway, NJ 08854-8020
Phone: (732) 445-2675
Web site: www.pharmacy.rutgers.edu

NEW MEXICO

College of Pharmacy
University of New Mexico
Health Sciences Center
2502 Marble NE
Albuquerque, NM 87131-5691
Phone: (505) 272-3241
Web site: www.hsc.unm.edu/pharmacy

NEW YORK

Arnold & Marie Schwartz College of Pharmacy and Health Sciences
Long Island University
75 DeKalb Avenue
Brooklyn, NY 11201
Phone: (718) 488-1234
Web site: www.liu.edu

College of Pharmacy and Allied Health Professions
St. John's University
8000 Utopia Parkway
Jamaica, NY 11439
Phone: (718) 990-1415
Web site: www.stjohns.edu

School of Pharmacy and Pharmaceutical Sciences
University at Buffalo
126 Cooke Hall
P.O. Box 601200
Buffalo NY 14260-1200
Phone: (716) 645-2823
Web site: www.pharmacy.buffalo.edu

Union University
Albany College of Pharmacy
106 New Scotland
Albany, NY 12208
Phone: (518) 445-7200
Web site: www.acp.edu

NORTH CAROLINA

School of Pharmacy
Campbell University
P.O. Box 1090
Science Building
Room 101
Buies Creek, NC 27506
Phone: (910) 893-1685
Web site: www.campbell.edu/pharmacy/ index.html

School of Pharmacy
Wingate University
P.O. Box 3087
Wingate, NC 28174-0159
Phone: (704) 233-8331
Web site: www.pharmacy.wingate.edu/home.asp

School of Pharmacy
University of North Carolina
Beard Hall, CB#7360
Chapel Hill, NC 27599-7360
Phone: (919) 966-1121
Web site: www.pharmacy.unc.edu

NORTH DAKOTA

College of Pharmacy
North Dakota State University
123 Sudro Hall
Fargo, ND 58105-5055
Phone: (701) 231-6469
Web site: www.ndsu.nodak.edu/pharmacy

OHIO

College of Pharmacy
Ohio Northern University
525 South Main
Ada, OH 45810
Phone: (419) 772-2275
Web site: www.onu.edu/pharmacy

College of Pharmacy
The Ohio State University
217 Parks Hall
500 West 12th Avenue
Columbus, OH 43210-1291
Phone: (614) 292-2266
Web site: www.pharmacy.ohio-state.edu

College of Pharmacy
University of Cincinnati
Medical Center
3223 Eden Avenue
P.O. Box 670004
Cincinnati, OH 45267-0004
Phone: (513) 558-3784
Web site: www.pharmacy.uc.edu

College of Pharmacy
The University of Toledo
2801 West Bancroft Street
Toledo, OH 43606-3390
Phone: (419) 530-1904
Web site: www.utpharmacy.org

OKLAHOMA

College of Pharmacy
Southwestern Oklahoma State University
100 Campus Drive
Weatherford, OK 73096
Phone: (580) 774-3105
Web site: www.swosu.edu/depts/pharmacy/index.htm

College of Pharmacy
University of Oklahoma
P.O. Box 26901
Oklahoma City, OK 73190
Phone: (405) 271-6484
Web site: www.oupharmacy.com

OREGON

College of Pharmacy
Oregon State University
203 Pharmacy Building
Corvallis, OR 97331-3507
Phone: (541) 737-3424
Web site: www.pharmacy.oregonstate.edu

PENNSYLVANIA

Mylan School of Pharmacy
Duquesne University
306 Bayer Learning Center
Pittsburgh, PA 15282
Phone: (412) 396-6380
Web site: www.pharmacy.duq.edu/LECOM

School of Pharmacy
Lake Erie College of Osteopathic Medicine
1858 West Grandview Boulevard
Erie, PA 16509-1025
Phone (814) 866-6641
Web site: www.lecom.edu/pharmacy

Philadelphia College of Pharmacy
University of the Sciences in Philadelphia
600 South 43rd Street
Philadelphia, PA 19104-4495
Phone: (215) 596-8870
Web site: www.usip.edu/academics/pharmacy.html

School of Pharmacy
Temple University
3307 North Broad Street
Philadelphia, PA 19140
Phone: (215) 707-4990
Web site: www.temple.edu/pharmacy

School of Pharmacy
University of Pittsburgh
1104 Salk Hall
Pittsburgh, PA 15261-1911
Phone: (412) 648-8579
Web site: www.pharmacy.pitt.edu

Nesbitt School of Pharmacy
Wilkes University
Wilkes-Barre, PA 18766
Phone: (570) 408-4280
Web site: www.pharmacy.wilkes.edu

PUERTO RICO

School of Pharmacy
University of Puerto Rico
P.O. Box 365067
San Juan, PR 00936-5067
Phone: (787) 758-2525
Web site: www.rcm.upr.edu/academics.html

RHODE ISLAND

College of Pharmacy
University of Rhode Island
41 Lower College Road
Fogerty Hall
Kingston, RI 02881-0809
Phone: (401) 874-2614
Web site: www.uri.edu/pharmacy

SOUTH CAROLINA

College of Pharmacy
Medical University of South Carolina
280 Calhoun Street
P.O. Box 250141
Charleston, SC 29425-2301
Phone: (843) 792-3115
Web site: www.musc.edu/pharmacy

College of Pharmacy
University of South Carolina
Columbia, SC 29208
Phone: (803) 777-4151
Web site: www.pharm.sc.edu

SOUTH DAKOTA

College of Pharmacy
South Dakota State University
Pharmacy Building, Room 125
P.O. Box 2202C
Brookings, SD 57007
Phone: (605) 688-6197
Web site: www3.sdstate.edu/academics/collegeofpharmacy

TENNESSEE

College of Pharmacy
University of Tennessee
847 Monroe Avenue, Suite 226
Memphis, TN 38163
Phone: (901) 448-6036
Web site: www.pharmacy.utmem.edu

TEXAS

College of Pharmacy and Health Sciences
Texas Southern University
3100 Cleburne
Houston, TX 77004
Phone: (713) 313-7164
Web site: www.tsu.edu/academics/pharmacy/index.asp

School of Pharmacy
Texas Tech University
Health Sciences Center
1300 South Coulter Street
Amarillo, TX 79106
Phone: (806) 354-5463
Web site: www.pharmacy.ama.ttuhsc.edu

College of Pharmacy
University of Houston
141 Science and Research
2 Building
Houston, TX 77204-5000
Phone: (713) 743-1300
Web site: www.uh.edu/pharmacy

College of Pharmacy
University of Texas at Austin
2409 University Avenue
Austin, TX 78712
Phone: (512) 471-3718
Web site: www.utexas.edu/pharmacy

UTAH

College of Pharmacy
University of Utah
30 South 2000
East Room 201
Salt Lake City, UT 84112-5820
Phone: (801) 581-6731
Web site: www.pharmacy.utah.edu

VIRGINIA

School of Pharmacy
Hampton University
Kittrell Hall
Hampton, VA 23668
Phone: (757) 727-5071
Web site: www.hamptonu.edu/pharm/index.htm

Bernard J. Dunn School of Pharmacy
Shenandoah University
1460 University Drive
Winchester, VA 22601
Phone: (540) 665-1282
Web site: www.pharmacy.su.edu

School of Pharmacy
Virginia Commonwealth University
MCV Campus
P.O. Box 980581
410 North 12th Street
Richmond, VA 23298-0581
Phone: (804) 828-3006
Web site: www.pharmacy.vcu.edu

WASHINGTON

School of Pharmacy
University of Washington
H-364 Health Science Building
P.O. Box 357631
Seattle, WA 98195
Phone: (206) 543-2030
Web site: www.pharmacy.washington.edu

College of Pharmacy
Washington State University
P.O. Box 646510
105 Wegner Hall
Pullman, WA 99164-6510
Phone: (509) 335-5901
Web site: www.pharmacy.wsu.edu

WEST VIRGINIA

School of Pharmacy
West Virginia University
Room 1136 HSN
Health Science Center
P.O. Box 9500
Morgantown, WV 26506-9500
Phone: (304) 293-5101
Web site: www.hsc.wvu.edu/sop

WISCONSIN

School of Pharmacy
University of Wisconsin—Madison
777 Highland Avenue
Madison, WI 53705-2222
Phone: (608) 262-1416
Web site: www.pharmacy.wisc.edu

WYOMING

School of Pharmacy
University of Wyoming
P.O. Box 3375
Laramie, WY 82071-3375
Phone: (307) 766-6120
Web site: www.uwyo.edu/pharmacy

State Boards
of Pharmacy

ALABAMA

Louise Foster Jones, Executive Secretary
10 Inverness Center, Suite 110
Birmingham, AL 35242
Phone: (205) 981-2280
Fax: (205) 981-2330
E-mail: ljones@albop.com
Web site: www.albop.com

ALASKA

Sher Zinn, Licensing Examiner
P.O. Box 110806
Juneau, AK 99811-0806
Phone: (907) 465-2589
Fax: (907) 465-2974
E-mail: sher_zinn@commerce.state.ak.us
Web site: www.commerce.state.ak.us/occ/ppha.htm

ARIZONA

Harlan "Hal" Wand, Executive Director
4425 W Olive Avenue, Suite 140
Glendale, AZ 85302-3844
Phone: (623) 463-2727
Fax: (623) 934-0583
E-mail: hwand@azsbp.com
Web site: www.pharmacy.state.az.us

ARKANSAS

Charles S. Campbell, Executive Director
101 East Capitol, Suite 218
Little Rock, AR 72201
Phone: (501) 682-0190
Fax: (501) 682-0195
E-mail: charlie.campbell@arkansas.gov
Web site: www.arkansas.gov/asbp

CALIFORNIA

Patricia F. Harris, Executive Officer
400 R Street, Suite 4070
Sacramento, CA 95814
Phone: (916) 445-5014
Fax: (916) 327-6308
E-mail: patricia_harris@dca.ca.gov
Web site: www.pharmacy.ca.gov

COLORADO

Susan L. Warren, Program Director
1560 Broadway, Suite 1310
Denver, CO 80202-5143
Phone: (303) 894-7800
Fax: (303) 894-7764
E-mail: susan.warren@dora.state.co.us
Web site: www.dora.state.co.us/pharmacy

CONNECTICUT

Michelle B. Sylvestre, Drug Control Agent and Board Administrator
165 Capitol Avenue
 State Office Building, Room 147
Hartford, CT 06106
Phone: (860) 713-6070
Fax: (860) 713-7242
E-mail: michelle.sylvestre@po.state.ct.us
Web site: www.ct.gov/dcp/site/default.asp

DELAWARE

David W. Dryden, Executive Secretary
Division of Professional Regulation
Cannon Building
861 Silver Lake Boulevard, Suite 203
Dover, DE 19904
Phone: (302) 744-4526
Fax: (302) 739-2711
E-mail: boardofpharmacy@state.de.us
Web site: www.dpr.delaware.gov

DISTRICT OF COLUMBIA

Bonnie Rampersaud, Executive Director
717 – 14th Street NW, Suite 600
Washington, DC 20005
Phone: (202) 724-4900
Fax: (202) 724-8471
E-mail: nathaniel.massaquoi@dc.gov
Web site: www.dchealth.dc.gov

FLORIDA

Rebecca Poston, Executive Director
4052 Bald Cypress Way, Bin# C04
Tallahassee, FL 32399-3254
Phone: (850) 245-4292
Fax: (850) 413-6982
E-mail: rebecca_poston@doh.state.fl.us

GEORGIA

Sylvia L. "Sandy" Bond, Executive Director
Professional Licensing Boards
237 Coliseum Drive
Macon, GA 31217-3858
Phone: (478) 207-1640
Fax: (478) 207-1660
E-mail: slbond@sos.state.ga.us
Web site: www.sos.state.ga.us/plb/pharmacy

HAWAII

Lee Ann Teshima, Executive Officer
P.O. Box 3469
Honolulu, HI 96801
Phone: (808) 586-2694
Fax: (808) 586-2874
E-mail: pharmacy@dcca.hawaii.gov
Web site: www.hawaii.gov/dcca/areas/pvl/boards/pharmacy

IDAHO

Richard K. "Mick" Markuson, Executive Director
3380 Americana Terrace, Suite 320
Boise, ID 83706
Phone: (208) 334-2356
Fax: (208) 334-3536
E-mail: rmarkuson@bop.state.id.us
Web site: www.accessidaho.org/bop

ILLINOIS

Kim Scott, Pharmacy Board Liaison
320 West Washington, 3rd Floor
Springfield, IL 62786
Phone: (217) 782-8556
Fax: (217) 782-7645
E-mail: PRFGROUP10@idfpr.com
Web site: www.idfpr.com

INDIANA

Joshua Bolin, Director
402 West Washington St., Room W072
Indianapolis, IN 46204-2739
Phone: (317) 234-2067
Fax: (317) 233-4236
E-mail: pla4@pla.in.gov
Web site: www.in.gov/pla/bandc/isbp

IOWA

Lloyd K. Jessen, Executive Director/Secretary
400 SW 8th Street, Suite E
Des Moines, IA 50309-4688
Phone: (515) 281-5944
Fax: (515) 281-4609
E-mail: lloyd.jessen@ibpe.state.ia.us
Web site: www.state.ia.us/ibpe

KANSAS

Debra L. Billingsley, Executive Secretary/Director
Landon State Office Building
900 Jackson, Room 560
Topeka, KS 66612-1231
Phone: (785) 296-4056
Fax: (785) 296-8420
E-mail: pharmacy@pharmacy.state.ks.us
Web site: www.accesskansas.org/pharmacy

KENTUCKY

Michael A. Burleson, Executive Director
23 Millcreek Park
Frankfort, KY 40601-9230
Phone: (502) 573-1580
Fax: (502) 573-1582
E-mail: mike.burleson@ky.gov
Web site: http://pharmacy.ky.gov

LOUISIANA

Malcolm J. Broussard, Executive Director
5615 Corporate Boulevard, Suite 8E
Baton Rouge, LA 70808-2537
Phone: (225) 925-6496
Fax: (225) 925-6499
E-mail: mbroussard@labp.com
Web site: www.labp.com

MAINE

Geraldine L. "Jeri" Betts, Board Administrator
Department of Professional/Financial Regulations
35 State House Station
Augusta, ME 04333
Phone: (207) 624-8689
Fax: (207) 624-8637
E-mail: geraldine.l.betts@maine.gov
Web site: www.maineprofessionalreg.org

MARYLAND

La Verne George Naesea, Executive Director
4201 Patterson Avenue
Baltimore, MD 21215-2299
Phone: (410) 764-4755
Fax: (410) 358-6207
E-mail: lnaesea@dhmh.state.md.us
Web site: www.dhmh.state.md.us/pharmacyboard

MASSACHUSETTS

Charles R. Young, Executive Director
239 Causeway Street, Room 216
Boston, MA 02114
Phone: (617) 973-0800
Fax: (617) 973-0983
E-mail: charles.young@state.ma.us
Web site: www.mass.gov/dpl/boards/ph/index.htm

MICHIGAN

Rae Ramsdell, Director
Licensing Division
611 West Ottawa, 1st Floor
P.O. Box 30670
Lansing, MI 48909-8170
Phone: (517) 335-0918
Fax: (517) 373-2179
E-mail: rhramsd@michigan.gov
Web site: www.michigan.gov/healthlicense

MINNESOTA

David E. Holmstrom, Executive Director
2829 University Avenue SE, Suite 530
Minneapolis, MN 55414-3251
Phone: (612) 617-2201
Fax: (612) 617-2212
E-mail: David.Holmstrom@state.mn.us
Web site: www.phcybrd.state.mn.us

MISSISSIPPI

Leland "Mac" McDivitt, Executive Director
204 Key Drive, Suite D
Madison, MS 39110
Phone: (601) 605-5388
Fax: (601) 605-9546
E-mail: lmcdivitt@mbp.state.ms.us
Web site: www.mbp.state.ms.us

MISSOURI

Kevin E. Kinkade, Executive Director
P.O. Box 625
Jefferson City, MO 65102
Phone: (573) 751-0091
Fax: (573) 526-3464
E-mail: kevin.kinkade@pr.mo.gov
Web site: www.pr.mo.gov/pharmacists.asp

MONTANA

Rebecca H. Deschamps, Executive Director
P.O. Box 200513
301 South Park Avenue, 4th Floor
Helena, MT 59620-0513
Phone: (406) 841-2355
Fax: (406) 841-2305
E-mail: dlibsdpha@state.mt.us

NEBRASKA

Becky Wisell, Executive Secretary
P.O. Box 94986
Lincoln, NE 68509-4986
Phone: (402) 471-2118
Fax: (402) 471-3577
E-mail: becky.wisell@hhss.ne.gov
Web site: www.hhs.state.ne.us

NEVADA

Larry Pinson, Executive Secretary
555 Double Eagle Court, Suite 1100
Reno, NV 89521
Phone: (775) 850-1440
Fax: (775) 850-1444
E-mail: pharmacy@govmail.state.nv.us
Web site: www.state.nv.us/pharmacy

NEW HAMPSHIRE

Paul G. Boisseau, Executive Secretary
57 Regional Drive
Concord, NH 03301-8518
Phone: (603) 271-2350
Fax: (603) 271-2856
E-mail: pharmacy.board@nh.gov
Web site: www.nh.gov/pharmacy

NEW JERSEY

Joanne Boyer, Executive Director
124 Halsey Street
Newark, NJ 07102
Phone: (973) 504-6450
Fax: (973) 648-3355
E-mail: boyerj@dca.lps.state.nj.us
Web site: www.state.nj.us/lps/ca/boards.htm

NEW MEXICO

William Harvey, Executive Director/Chief Drug Inspector
5200 Oakland NE, Suite A
Albuquerque, NM 87113
Phone: (505) 222-9830
Fax: (505) 222-9845
E-mail: william.harvey@state.nm.us
Web site: www.state.nm.us/pharmacy

NEW YORK

Lawrence H. Mokhiber, Executive Secretary
89 Washington Avenue, 2nd Floor West
Albany, NY 12234-1000
Phone: (518) 474-3817 ext 130
Fax: (518) 473-6995
E-mail: pharmbd@mail.nysed.gov
Web site: www.op.nysed.gov

NORTH CAROLINA

David R. Work, Executive Director
P.O. Box 4560
Chapel Hill, NC 27515-4560
Phone: (919) 942-4454
Fax: (919) 967-5757
E-mail: drw@ncbop.org
Web site: www.ncbop.org

NORTH DAKOTA

Howard C. Anderson Jr., Executive Director
P.O. Box 1354
Bismarck, ND 58502-1354
Phone: (701) 328-9535
Fax: (701) 328-9536
E-mail: ndboph@btinet.net
Web site: www.nodakpharmacy.com

OHIO

William T. Winsley, Executive Director
77 South High Street, Room 1702
Columbus, OH 43215-6126
Phone: (614) 466-4143
Fax: (614) 752-4836
E-mail: exec@bop.state.oh.us
Web site: www.pharmacy.ohio.gov

OKLAHOMA

Bryan H. Potter, Executive Director
4545 Lincoln Boulevard, Suite 112
Oklahoma City, OK 73105-3488
Phone: (405) 521-3815
Fax: (405) 521-3758
E-mail: pharmacy@pharmacy.ok.gov
Web site: www.pharmacy.ok.gov

OREGON

Gary A. Schnabel, Executive Director
800 NE Oregon Street, Suite 425
Portland, OR 97232
Phone: (971) 673-0001
Fax: (971) 673-0002
E-mail: pharmacy.board@state.or.us
Web site: www.pharmacy.state.or.us

PENNSYLVANIA

Melanie A. Zimmerman, Executive Secretary
P.O. Box 2649
Harrisburg, PA 17105-2649
Phone: (717) 783-7156
Fax: (717) 787-7769
E-mail: st-pharmacy@state.pa.us
Web site: www.dos.state.pa.us/pharm

PUERTO RICO

Magda Bouet, Executive Director
Department of Health, Board of Pharmacy
Call Box 10200
Santurce, PR 00908
Phone: (787) 724-7282
Fax: (787) 725-7903
E-mail: mbouet@salud.gov.pr

RHODE ISLAND

Catherine A. Cordy, Executive Director
3 Capitol Hill, Room 205
Providence, RI 02908-5097
Phone: (401) 222-2837
Fax: (401) 222-2158
E-mail: cathyc@doh.state.ri.us
Web site: www.health.ri.gov/hsr/professions/pharmacy.php

SOUTH CAROLINA

Lee Ann Bundrick, Administrator
Kingstree Bldg.
110 Centerview Drive, Suite 306
Columbia, SC 29210
Phone: (803) 896-4700
Fax: (803) 896-4596
E-mail: bundricl@llr.sc.gov
Web site: www.llronline.com/POL/pharmacy

SOUTH DAKOTA

Dennis M. Jones, Executive Secretary
4305 South Louise Avenue, Suite 104
Sioux Falls, SD 57106
Phone: (605) 362-2737
Fax: (605) 362-2738
E-mail: dennis.jones@state.sd.us
Web site: www.state.sd.us/doh/pharmacy

TENNESSEE

Kendall M. Lynch, Director
500 James Robertson Parkway, 2nd Floor
Davy Crockett Tower
Nashville, TN 37243-1149
Phone: (615) 741-2718
Fax: (615) 741-2722
E-mail: Kendall.Lynch@state.tn.us
Web site: www.state.tn.us/commerce/boards/pharmacy

TEXAS

Gay Dodson, Executive Director
333 Guadalupe
Tower 3, Suite 600
Austin, TX 78701-3942
Phone: (512) 305-8000
Fax: (512) 305-8082
E-mail: gay.dodson@tsbp.state.tx.us
Web site: www.tsbp.state.tx.us

UTAH

Diana L. Baker, Bureau Manager
P.O. Box 146741
Salt Lake City, UT 84114-6741
Phone: (801) 530-6179
Fax: (801) 530-6511
E-mail: dbaker@utah.gov
Web site: www.dopl.utah.gov

VERMONT

Peggy Atkins, Board Administrator
Office of Professional Regulation
26 Terrace Street, Drawer 09
Montpelier, VT 05609-1106
Phone: (802) 828-2373
Fax: (802) 828-2465
E-mail: patkins@sec.state.vt.us
Web site: www.vtprofessionals.org

VIRGINIA

Elizabeth Scott Russell, Executive Director
6603 West Broad Street, 5th Floor
Richmond, VA 23230-1712
Phone: (804) 662-9911
Fax: (804) 662-9313
E-mail: scotti.russell@dhp.virginia.gov
Web site: www.dhp.state.va.us/pharmacy/default.htm

WASHINGTON

Steven M. Saxe, Executive Director
P.O. Box 47863
Olympia, WA 98504-7863
Phone: (360) 236-4825
Fax: (360) 586-4359
E-mail: Steven.Saxe@doh.wa.gov
Web site: https://fortress.wa.gov/doh/hpqa1/HPS4/Pharmacy/default.htm

WEST VIRGINIA

William T. Douglass Jr., Executive Director and General Counsel
232 Capitol Street
Charleston, WV 25301
Phone: (304) 558-0558
Fax: (304) 558-0572
E-mail: wdouglass@wvbop.com
Web site: www.wvbop.com

WISCONSIN

Tom Ryan, Bureau Director
1400 East Washington
P.O. Box 8935
Madison, WI 53708-8935
Phone: (608) 266-2811
Fax: (608) 267-0644
E-mail: thomas.ryan@drl.state.wi.us
Web site: www.drl.state.wi.us

WYOMING

James T. Carder, Executive Director
632 South David Street
Casper, WY 82601
Phone: (307) 234-0294
Fax: (307) 234-7226
E-mail: jcarde@state.wy.us
Web site: http://pharmacyboard.state.wy.us

Licensure Requirements

INTERN LICENSE

Upon registration in a pharmacy college/school, students are eligible to become pharmacy interns. Because some states require that interns be licensed, check with the dean's office of your college/school concerning internship requirements in your state. All states require a minimum of 1,500 internship hours under the guidance of a pharmacy preceptor licensed in the state in which the student is registered. These hours may be obtained during summer breaks between professional years in the college of pharmacy, breaks during the academic year, or after graduation. Although some state boards of pharmacy require that a minimum number of these hours be obtained after graduation, the current trend is to complete the hours beforehand so that you can take the state board of pharmacy examination to become licensed on graduation.

A number of boards of pharmacy give students credit for the entire 1,500 hours of internship during the clinical curriculum of a college/school of pharmacy. Some boards of pharmacy give only 400 hours, whereas other boards recognize the clinical experience in the Pharm.D. program for the entire internship-hour requirements.

PHARMACY LICENSE REQUIREMENTS

After graduation, you must take a theoretical and practical examination administered by a state board of pharmacy. The National Association of Boards of Pharmacy's standardized North American Pharmacist Licensure Examination™ (NAPLEX)® is administered by all state boards of pharmacy, with the exception of California. (California conducts its own licensure examination.) The NAPLEX is administered several times a year; each state board adheres to a standardized set of dates for giving the examination. These dates can be obtained from each state board of pharmacy office.

NAPLEX®

One of the most important functions of boards of pharmacy is to protect the public health and welfare. Each state board must set standards of competence for the practice of pharmacy. State laws require the assessment of the proficiency of each candidate in the knowledge, skills, and abilities necessary for the practice of pharmacy.

State boards use the NAPLEX® to make that assessment. A candidate for licensure who passes this examination is judged to have the required proficiency in that state and can also practice pharmacy in other licensing jurisdictions that offer reciprocity.

The licensing examination, which is oriented toward professional practice, is a qualifying evaluation rather than a competitive test. The NAPLEX® Review Committee established standards of knowledge, skills, and abilities they consider essential for the practice of pharmacy. NAPLEX® is used to assess these standards and is one determinant of a candidate's qualification for licensure. By nature, the examination emphasizes that facts and information are meaningless without the ability to apply them in a practical situation. Furthermore, it highlights skills and abilities that must be maintained throughout the candidate's professional career.

The NAPLEX® is a computer-adaptive test used by the state boards of pharmacy as part of their assessment of a candidate's competence to practice pharmacy. It consists of 185 multiple-choice test questions. A total of 150 questions are used to calculate your test score, while the other thirty-five items are pretest questions that do not affect your NAPLEX® score. The questions cover all aspects of pharmacy, with a majority of the questions asked in a scenario-based format (i.e., patient profiles with accompanying test questions). The examination is administered three times per year in January, June, and October at specific computer centers across the country.

RECIPROCITY BETWEEN STATES

Reciprocity is the process of transferring a license from one state to another. Most states recognize test scores from other states with some exceptions, such as California, which requires pharmacists to take its own board of pharmacy examination before becoming licensed. Typically, on completing the state board of pharmacy requirements of a particular state, you must practice one year before being able to reciprocate your license in another state. Although each state law is different, many states participate in the score transfer program, which transfers the NAPLEX® test scores to another state.